MW00637314

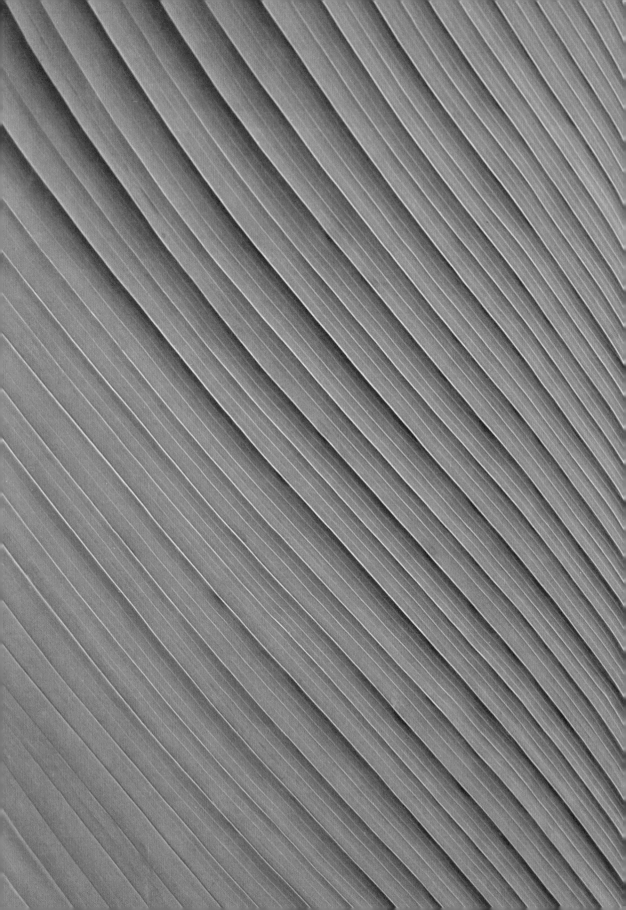

Praise for *Well to the Core*

I first encountered Robin's work several years ago, during a stretch of time when I felt disconnected from my body and in need of a guide back to myself. Robin taught me practices and perspectives that helped put me on a path toward health in body and spirit. I know these beautiful pages will do that same gentle guiding work for so many people.

SHAUNA NIEQUIST
New York Times bestselling author

A healthy balance of physical and mental health is essential for every parent. In *Well to the Core*, Robin's "grace-over-guilt" mentality, coupled with her vast knowledge of living a balanced lifestyle, inspires and encourages readers to be more of who they were meant to be.

AMY MCCREADY
Founder of Positive Parenting Solutions and author of *The "Me, Me, Me" Epidemic*

Beautifully weaving together personal stories with research-backed tips and insights, *Well to the Core* provides a road map for anyone who'd like to take the first step toward health and wellness. In this practical guide, Robin Long gently invites you to consider and rethink what it means to be healthy, from the inside out.

DR. ANDREA GURNEY
Psychologist, professor, and author of *Reimagining Your Love Story*

Live your best life with *Well to the Core*! Robin has written the book we've all been craving: an expert guidebook for long-lasting health and well-being. With seasoned expertise, Robin helps us choose grace over guilt and see that vibrant health is possible. Get ready for an energizing, freeing experience digging into these practical and inspiring pages. I highly recommend this incredible book!

LARA CASEY
Author of *Make It Happen* and *Cultivate*

Robin's "grace over guilt" mentality is at the heart of everything she does—and it has transformed the way I think about wellness. *Well to the Core* provides an inspiring overview of a much-needed perspective shift around healthy living. You're going to love this transformative book!

REBEKAH LYONS
Bestselling author of *Rhythms of Renewal*

What Lindywell Members Are Saying

I've had health issues off and on my entire adult life, and back issues since I was sixteen years old. I've focused a lot on my health and wellness and fought hard to accept my body for what it is. Pilates and Robin's positive talk have helped me to stop seeing my body as the enemy.

    EMILY B.

I can honestly say I have never been this consistent with any kind of workout— and not only have I been consistent, but I have actually found something that I enjoy doing! I look forward to my daily Pilates time and have even chosen to do a workout for an energy boost when I notice that I'm feeling sluggish.

    KRISTEN W.

As a mom of four, I don't always find it easy to get time for myself. But fifteen minutes of Pilates is attainable and so satisfying to know that I'm doing something for me. I can definitely recognize the days I have done Pilates and the days that I've missed. The benefits of Pilates continue even after leaving the mat.

    CARMEN W.

The Lindywell approach—only fifteen minutes a day, and grace over guilt— and the variety of routines available are key for me. Lindywell has helped me discipline myself in my exercise, and that self-disciple has spilled over into other areas of my life!

    BECKI A.

Everything Robin stands for and teaches is exactly what I need: grace over guilt, trust the process—her workouts are helping me become not only physically healthy but mentally healthy as well. This program is changing me from the inside out.

    HOLLY P.

The first time I tried Pilates, I was in awe of the way my body felt after the class. I love Robin and Lindywell, the support of the other members, and the opportunity to share our triumphs as well as the days we feel more like a rock than a rock star. This investment in myself is the best money I've ever spent.

MARY L.

Lindywell has radically changed my health. I was a collegiate athlete, and I enjoy being active. However, over the years, I've found it difficult to motivate myself to go to the gym or be a part of workout groups due to my busy schedule. Lindywell has completely changed how I approach fitness, and it has helped my mental health as well!

ALLIE B.

I joined Lindywell a year ago and recently had my annual physical. My blood work and blood pressure were all the best they've been in years. My doctor said I looked fantastic. It was great to get such affirmation and inspiration to keep giving it my best every day!

VICKIE J.

I have recovered strength in both body and mind through Robin's approach. Not only does Pilates heal the body; it also focuses and soothes the mind. I love the mind work it provides as much as I appreciate the body conditioning. And no scale can measure that.

DONNA M.

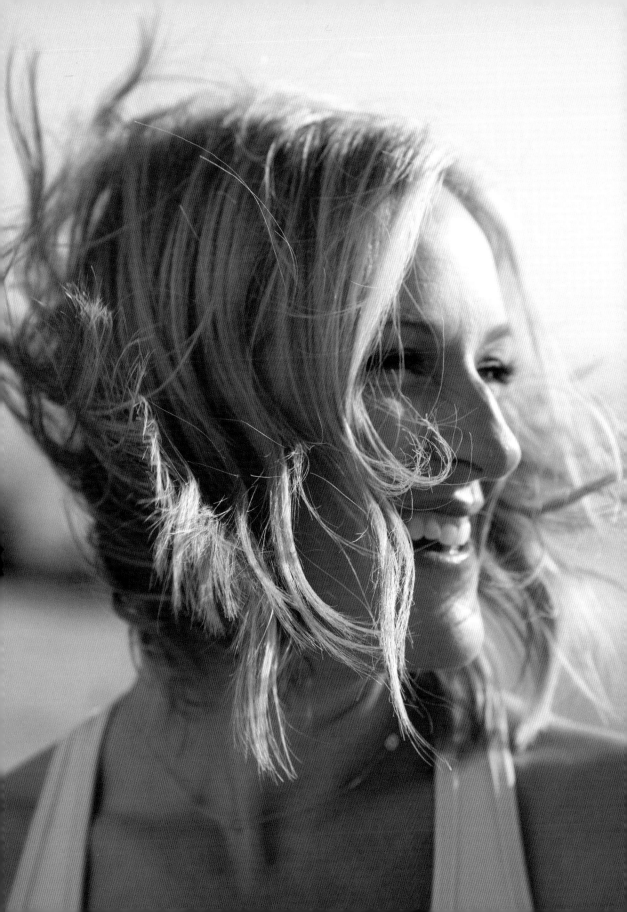

well to the core

ROBIN LONG

A Realistic, Guilt-Free Approach to Getting Fit
& Feeling Good for a Lifetime

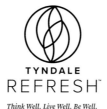

TYNDALE
REFRESH™

Think Well. Live Well. Be Well.

MEDICAL DISCLAIMER

The health, wellness, fitness, and nutritional information in this book is designed for educational purposes only. This information should not be relied on as a substitute for professional medical advice, diagnosis, or treatment. If you have any concerns or questions about your health, consult with a physician or other health care professional. Always consult your physician or health care provider before beginning a new exercise or nutrition program.

Visit Tyndale online at tyndale.com.

Visit Robin online at lindywell.com.

Tyndale and Tyndale's quill logo are registered trademarks of Tyndale House Ministries. *Tyndale Refresh* and the Tyndale Refresh logo are trademarks of Tyndale House Ministries. Tyndale Refresh is a nonfiction imprint of Tyndale House Publishers, Carol Stream, Illinois.

Well to the Core: A Realistic, Guilt-Free Approach to Getting Fit and Feeling Good for a Lifetime

Designed by Libby Dykstra

Edited by Stephanie Rische

Published in association with Jenni Burke of Illuminate Literary Agency: www.illuminateliterary.com.

For information about special discounts for bulk purchases, please contact Tyndale House Publishers at csresponse@tyndale.com, or call 1-855-277-9400.

Library of Congress Cataloging-in-Publication Data

A catalog record for this book is available from the Library of Congress.

ISBN 978-1-4964-7262-5

Printed in China

29	28	27	26	25	24	23
7	6	5	4	3	2	1

For my family:
I am forever grateful for your
unconditional love and support.

For the Lindywell community:
You inspire me and encourage me every single day.
Thank you for being part of this movement. We're in
this together, and I could not do this without you.

contents

Introduction 1

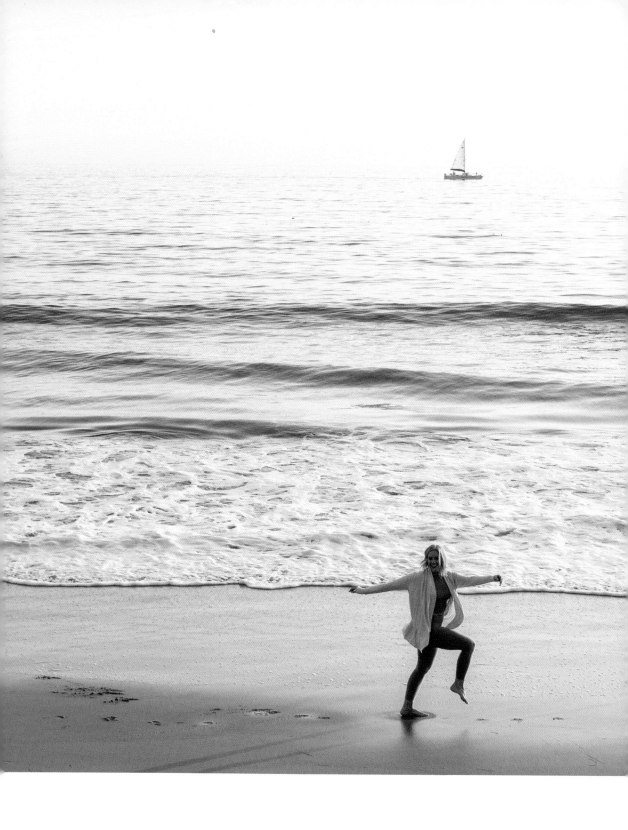

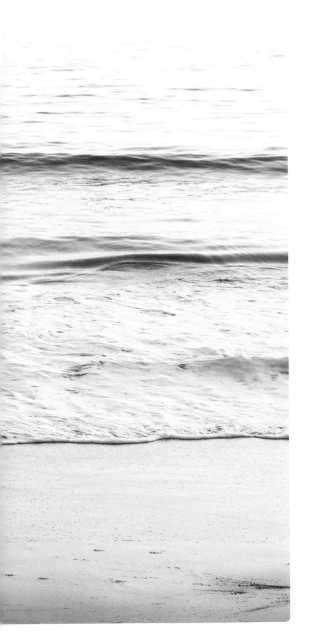

Introduction

I remember the moment clearly. I was eight years old, crying under a pinball machine in my friend Kayla's basement. As I heard her coming down the stairs to find me, I did my best to stop the tears.

We'd spent the day playing hide-and-seek, braiding our hair, dressing in matching outfits, and playing the way free-spirited young girls do. But as I wiped my tears under the pinball machine, my little spirit didn't feel so free anymore.

A few minutes earlier, we'd skipped outside in matching black spandex shorts and T-shirts tied with scrunchies to show my friend's parents how cute we looked as twins. While we stood in front of them awaiting their "oohs" and "aahs," her dad turned to her mom and said, "Wow, look how much skinnier Kayla's legs are than Robin's."

In that moment, my heart sank.

At eight years old, I was just beginning to notice the ways my body was different from my friends' bodies and how my thighs were bigger and rounder than those of the girls with stick-straight legs. That comment from my friend's dad pierced my heart and confirmed an emerging belief in my young mind: my body was bigger, and bigger was bad. My body was on display, and people were watching.

Decades later, here I am remembering that one tiny moment and still recovering from years of hating (and hiding) my thighs.

Of course, this wasn't the sole event that led to years of struggle with my body image. There have been other piercing moments that confirmed my insecurities. Like when I was trying on costumes for a dance performance, and my calves were too big to fit in the go-go boots. The other girls easily slipped their feet in, while the choreographer got onto her hands and knees to force my legs in, squeezing my calves and stretching the fabric to get the zipper up. Or when I was walking down the hallway of my college dormitory and I overheard a guy I was dating say I had a chin like Jay Leno's. While these were not life-defining moments, they stung, and they formed an inner narrative that affirmed my insecurities for years.

I'm willing to bet you've had similar moments in your life, even if the specifics of your story are different from mine. While working with thousands of women as a Pilates instructor and as the founder of Lindywell, a global Pilates, health, and wellness company, I've discovered that somewhere along the way, we've all internalized false messages about our bodies, ourselves, and our worth that stick with us throughout the years.

The Lies We've Been Taught

I'm lucky to have grown up in a loving, supportive home where my parents didn't put significant pressure on me to look a certain way or be a certain size. (Thank you, Mom and Dad!) And yet for most of my life, I struggled with body image and my relationship with food and exercise. I find this fascinating (and deeply concerning, as a mom of four young kids). My home was full of love and confidence-boosting messages, and my body shape was not far from the cultural "ideal," yet I still spent an unreasonable amount of time and energy wishing I looked different. I spent many years restricting my food intake through fad diets, exercising to work off

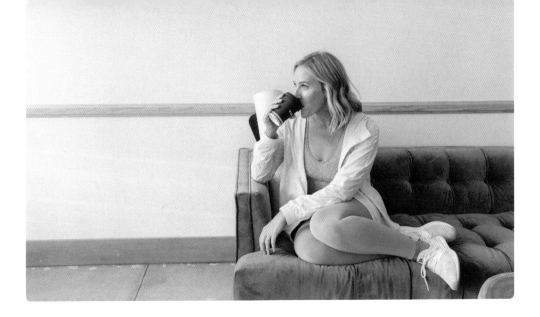

what I ate, and comparing my body to other women's bodies as a measure of my success, worth, and value. And if I'm not careful, I'm still tempted to do that today.

So if this pressure to look a certain way wasn't coming from my home and my family of origin, where did it come from?

The answer: everywhere else.

From a young age, women are taught to believe that our worth is measured by the size and shape of our bodies. Ads portray how happy we'll be when we lose weight, reduce cellulite, or finally get that lean, toned bikini body. Back in the day, magazines sucked us in with messages about how much celebrities ate in a day or how they "bounced back" after pregnancy. Now we are bombarded by online articles and social media images that try to convince us that if we would just eat and exercise a certain way, we would achieve the ideal look and lifestyle. We spend hours each day peeking at the highlight reels of other people's lives, all through the lens of filters and body-altering editing apps that have a subtle yet powerful impact on our self-image.

Movies and media depict beauty as a singular body type—a type that doesn't represent the many sizes and shapes of actual women.

From a young age, we're surrounded by comments like these:

"Oh, I shouldn't eat that."

"I really need to lose that baby weight."

"I'm never going to be ready for swimsuit season."

*True wellness doesn't come from
a number on a scale, the size of your waist,
or the absence of cellulite.*

From a young age, we hear women complimenting one another on their physical appearance, with a frequent focus on the size and shape of their bodies. We're taught that we need to change what we see in the mirror in order to be successful, fulfilled, relevant, and accepted. We think we have to punish our bodies with grueling exercise and harshly restrict our diets in order to reach an idealized size. We believe that if we just work hard enough, muster up more willpower, and hit some elusive "goal weight," we'll finally be healthier. And happier.

There's a Better Way

But what if the "rules" we've been sold by the diet and fitness industry don't actually work? What if happiness, health, and vitality aren't always found on the other side of losing ten pounds or slimming the size of your thighs?

If you're reading this book, it's safe to assume that you want to improve your health and get in shape. And that's a good thing—taking care of your health and improving the way you feel in your body is important. But many of us have confused taking care of our health with obsessing over our weight. There's a better way to reclaim your health, your fitness, and your body—an approach that is free of guilt and full of freedom. I wrote this book for every woman who is fed up with diet culture. It's for women who are tired of spending their mental capacity worrying, stressing, feeling bad about their bodies, and allowing lies of what they "should" be doing or how they should look to consume their precious time and energy.

I know how exhausting this is, because I used to live that way too. I wrote this book for women who want to take control of their health and feel their best but are tired of being at war with their bodies.

This book was born out of the work I've done with thousands of women all over the world. Over the past thirteen years as a Pilates instructor and as the CEO of a wellness company with the mission of helping every woman live life to the fullest, I've come to realize just how common the struggle is to care for our health. And this is a struggle I know all too well. I've weathered years of putting my health on the back burner, restricting my food intake, carrying multiple pregnancies, navigating grief and pregnancy loss, trying every exercise plan imaginable, struggling with anxiety, and trying (and failing at) more diets than I can even count. After years of struggle, I made it my mission to find a better way—and I now spend my days helping other women do the same.

In this book, we're shifting the conversation away from rules, fads, and trends that leave us feeling lost and confused, and toward what it truly means to be well in body, mind, and soul.

True wellness doesn't come from a number on a scale, the size of your waist, or the absence of cellulite. True wellness is found when you live out your purpose, enjoy all that life has to offer, and break free from the mental prison of stressing about what you're eating, how much you're exercising, or how much weight you need to lose in order to really start living.

It's possible to pursue a healthy lifestyle in a way that is guilt-free, realistic, and enjoyable. You can let go of the rules and myths about wellness you've been led to believe over the years. You can release the pressure you've been carrying all this time and exhale, knowing it's possible to make progress toward your goals, improve your fitness, and experience more wellness—without obsessing over numbers, neglecting what your body truly needs, or comparing yourself to others. You can embrace an approach that's free from guilt and shame, and full of compassion,

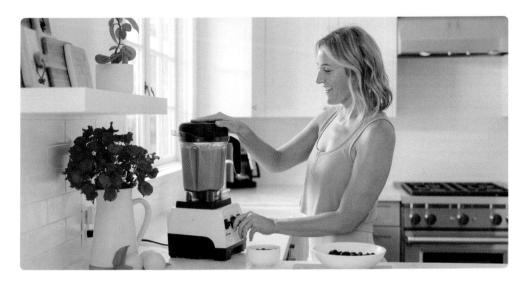

connection, and intention. As you do, you will redefine the way you look at fitness, food, and yourself for your entire lifetime.

The goal is to feel good—not just in your body but in your whole being. The next generation of girls deserves to be surrounded by and led by women who change the narrative so many of us grew up with. The tides are turning, and when we embrace a holistic approach to health and wellness, there's hope for the future. As our individual lives change, this shift will create lasting ripple effects for our families and our communities.

It starts with us. It starts with you.

The Ten Core Components

There are ten core components of wellness that will help you pursue a well-rounded, effective, and realistic approach to health. As you follow these principles, you can show up as the healthiest, most vibrant version of yourself and live your life to the fullest. These are the ten components:

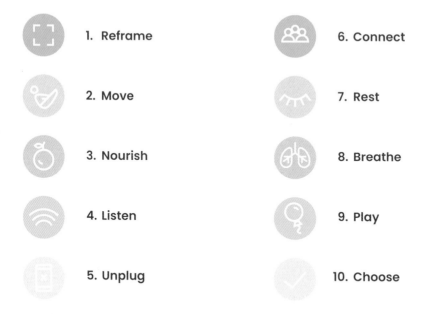

1. Reframe
2. Move
3. Nourish
4. Listen
5. Unplug
6. Connect
7. Rest
8. Breathe
9. Play
10. Choose

These components aren't intended to add more stress or work to your day; instead, they make your life easier. They serve as a sustainable and enjoyable road map toward better mental and physical health.[1] The goal is to care for ourselves from the inside out—it's not just about appearance but about truly being well to the core.

Each of the ten components can be implemented wherever you are on your journey toward health. I encourage you to start where you're at, with what you have.

You are not alone on your journey—you are surrounded by a whole community of women who are walking a similar path and facing similar challenges. A life of freedom and wellness is waiting for you, so let's begin!

---

[1] While wellness is absolutely impacted by the choices we make, it's also affected by our circumstances. This book would be incomplete if I didn't acknowledge the fact that there are disparities when it comes to basic elements of health, such as access to quality food, health care, and working conditions. Studies show that women are at a disadvantage in a variety of ways and that women of color, women with disabilities, and other marginalized groups face more challenges than others. In writing this book, I've attempted to provide tools and resources that are accessible to the widest group possible, while acknowledging that I write from a position of privilege in many ways.

Chapter 1

reframe

> How we think not only affects our own spirit, soul, and body but also people around us.
>
> Caroline Leaf

If you were to take a peek in my cupboards and refrigerator when I was a young adult, they would have revealed a spread of low-fat diet foods: sugar-free chocolate pudding, microwavable weight-loss meals, fat-free yogurt, and diet soda.

I was generally a happy and confident teen, and I spent most afternoons and weekends playing sports or dancing. But underneath the surface, I struggled with my body image. I never felt thin enough or fit enough, and I spent a good deal of time and energy trying to change the way my body looked. I forced myself to exercise (even

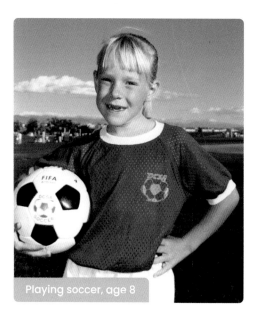
Playing soccer, age 8

after hours of dancing in the studio), restricted my calories, and had mental lists of good foods and bad foods.

I treasured my celebrity gossip magazines, hoping for inspiration and shortcuts to achieve the ideal body I so desired. Every magazine cover promised to reveal a secret that would give me the answers I was looking for. They were empty promises, however. This never-ending journey left me continually disappointed and frustrated with myself.

I was obsessed with the idea of losing weight; I didn't understand what it meant to be truly healthy, in body and mind. I thought being healthy was equivalent to being thin. In my quest for thinness, I was completely out of balance. Either I was overeating and struggling with motivation or I was trying to make up for those habits by frenetically burning calories or starting a new diet to get myself back on track once and for all. I constantly read diet books, bought every fat-free food I could find, and even used "metabolism-boosting" pills that left me shaky, queasy, and anxious.

When I was in college, I hit rock bottom. After many years of going on pendulum swings with my diet and exercise regimen, while being plagued by a persistent desire to lose weight and have a good body, I found myself in a dark place. Not only was I regularly binge drinking and binge eating late at night, but my sense of fulfillment was at an all-time low. I was discouraged and exhausted by the constant battle taking place inside me.

During my sophomore year of college, after returning home from a night out with friends—yet another evening of partying and bingeing on late-night pizza—I finally decided that something needed to change. I was so unhappy with myself. I was no longer having fun with the party scene, my friendships felt empty, and I knew deep down that this was not how I wanted to live. I knew there was more to life than the depressing cycle of drinking, bingeing, and trying to work it all off in the gym. I was weary of obsessing over how my body looked.

I realized that my environment and lifestyle weren't helping me move toward the kind of person I wanted to be. I was living a life I wasn't proud of, and I felt lost, helpless, stuck, and unhappy. But I wasn't sure how to shift the thoughts, habits, and patterns that were ruling my life and eroding my health and happiness.

On a cold, dreary Colorado night in my tiny college apartment, I dropped to my knees and prayed for the first time in a long time. I didn't have any profound words; I simply asked God to show me a way out. I was desperate.

Nothing magical happened that night, but I was open to seeing if God would really come through. One week later, I went home for winter break. We gathered with our extended family, as we usually did, for a night of appetizers and games on Christmas Eve. My cousin Mike and his wife, Angie, were in town. They were a few years older than I was, and I looked up to them as role models. They lived in California, wore cool clothes, had high-powered careers, and lived an exciting life.

As Angie and I were catching up over chocolate-covered Ritz Crackers and spinach artichoke dip, I shared my stress and inner struggles. I expected the typical response: "That's just college. You can do it; it will get better." But she surprised me by saying, "I'm actually in desperate need of a nanny. Maybe you could come live with us and take the time you need to figure it out."

What? Drop out of college and move to California? I thought.

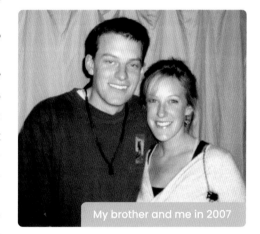

My brother and me in 2007

While it seemed far-fetched, I knew deep down that this was the answer to my prayer—this was my chance for a fresh start. While my parents were a bit hesitant about my decision to quit college without a plan to return, they ultimately supported me.

One week later, I dropped out of college, told my best friend I was moving out (one of the hardest conversations I'd had up to that point in my life), and packed up my bags. Then, with my brother by my side for moral support, I drove west in my little black Acura RSX.

That decision changed my life forever. Not only did it begin a new chapter for me, but it also provided an opportunity for me to transform my relationship with my body, food, and fitness. I wasn't just moving to another state; I was deciding to take control over my life.

While it's true that I eventually made changes to what I ate and how I exercised, and while these new routines helped me feel healthier and stronger, that wasn't where the changes started. The most important change I made was inside of me.

Change the Way You Think

The way we think about health, fitness, and our bodies matters. Our thoughts affect our actions, which means we can't change our lives until we change the way we think. So the first step to a more balanced approach is to become aware of beliefs that are keeping us stuck.

You may be wondering what you should eat or how many days a week you need to work out in order to experience transformation. But those aren't the most important questions to ask. Instead, we must reframe the way we think in order to create changes that last.

Here are five important reframes that I've developed through my own journey and as I've worked with thousands of women throughout my career. We'll revisit these new ways of thinking in the chapters ahead.

Reframe #1: Wellness Does Not Always Equal Weight Loss

Over the years, the diet and fitness industry has led us to believe that weight loss and good health are one and the same. As a result, we make decisions we *think* are good for our health, when in fact they are just about losing weight.

For years, I stocked my kitchen with low-fat, sugar-free, calorie-free diet food, believing I was making healthier choices. It turns out I was filling my body with processed garbage that wreaked havoc on my hormones, increased my cravings, and decreased my metabolism. While I successfully reduced my calorie and fat intake, the foods I was eating did not provide the nourishment I needed to thrive.

True wellness is being healthy in body and mind. The number on the scale is just one small part of a much larger picture, and research backs this truth.[1] You can be in great shape and wearing your ideal size of jeans while wreaking havoc on your mental health in the process. You can have a healthy BMI while lacking essential vitamins and nutrients that are central to keeping your body in balance. You can be getting in your cardio but so consumed by stress that your body is suffering. A

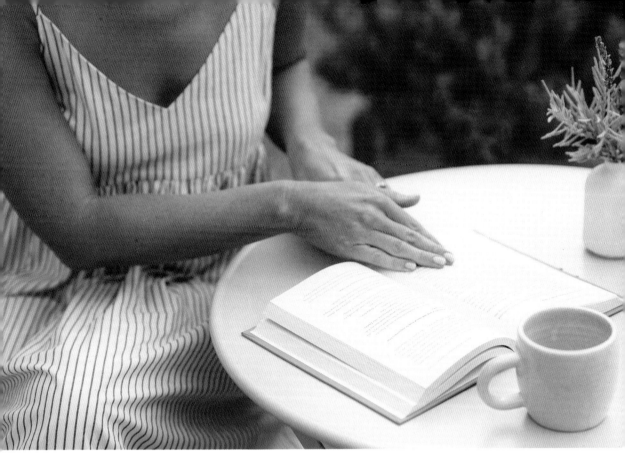

variety of factors determine our wellness—everything from the foods we eat to the stress we carry to the relationships we cultivate to the way we rest to the quality of our breathing to the health of our minds and spirits.[2]

It's time to break free from false patterns and pursue wellness as a holistic endeavor—one that goes far beyond weight loss as the ultimate goal and takes our entire well-being into account.

Reframe #2: It Doesn't Have to Be All or Nothing

One of the common misconceptions about diet and exercise is that you have to be all in or you might as well quit trying altogether. If any of the following viewpoints or actions resonate with you, you might be operating from this all-or-nothing mindset:

- You're either on or off a diet or exercise plan.

- You believe exercise must be long/hard/sweaty/exhausting to be worth it.

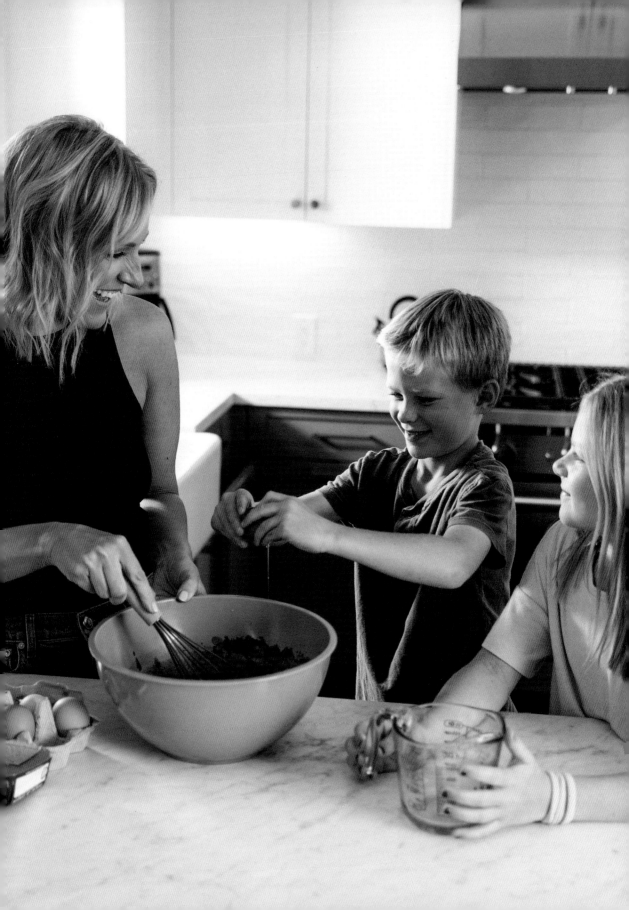

- You start a diet but give up when you can't follow it perfectly.
- You start a new exercise routine but throw in the towel after you skip a few workouts.
- When you indulge in an off-limits treat, you figure the whole day is a waste, so you keep indulging.

This all-or-nothing mindset kept me stuck for years. I would jump on a new diet fad or throw myself into a new workout program, only to get burned out in a few weeks and then give up. When it comes to making healthy choices, middle ground is hard to find. Life happens, and when we skip a workout and go off our eating plan, we often feel like we've failed. After this occurs a few times in a row (which, by the way, is a normal human experience), we throw in the towel altogether. Weeks pass as we consider ourselves "off the wagon" until we can muster the energy and motivation to start again, which may take days, weeks, months, or even years.

If this pattern sounds familiar, you're not alone—and it's not your fault.

Most diet and fitness programs measure success by how well you can stick to the plan—and some go so far as to send us guilt-inducing messages or notifications to let us know when we're not measuring up! We've been led to believe that we can start a diet on Monday and our lives will change by Friday, or that the hottest new fitness equipment or diet pill will transform our bodies once and for all.

Many women spend thousands of dollars on diets, pills, shakes, or programs. The diet industry is a $128 billion industry, yet the majority of people who go on diets don't succeed.[3] Clearly, diet companies are benefiting from this approach more than we are.

When success is defined by our ability to perfectly stick to a plan or make good decisions without leaving room for the constantly changing realities of daily life, it's nearly impossible to feel successful. When we recognize this all-or-nothing tendency, we'll be able to start reframing the way we think and discover a life of balance, grace, and self-compassion.

The truth is, a healthy lifestyle is not all or nothing. Every little bit counts when it comes to wellness. Research shows that ten minutes of exercise is better than zero minutes of exercise, one serving of veggies is better than zero servings of veggies, and five minutes in nature is better than none. You don't have to follow a strict set of rules to be the healthy and vibrant woman you want to be.

Once you make this shift, you start to recognize that perfection isn't required to make progress.

Reframe #3: Success and Failure Are Not Defined by Outward Appearance

In the same way that success is not defined by our ability to make perfect choices or stick to a plan perfectly, it's also not defined by outward appearance—despite what we may have been led to believe from a young age. As long as success is defined by the size of our jeans, the number on the scale, or the visibility of cellulite, we will miss out on what it truly means to be well.

Just because we've believed something for years doesn't mean it's true. Let me pause and say that again: just because we've believed something for years doesn't mean it's true.

I used to believe being thin always equaled being healthy. I also believed that smaller thighs would lead to greater happiness. But over the years, I've redefined what success looks like as it relates to health and wellness.

For me, success is getting dressed without falling into a spiral of negative thoughts about the way I look.

Success is putting on a swimsuit and jumping in the pool instead of hiding under a cover-up out of fear of what others might think.

Success is listening to my body and honoring its needs so I can live my life to the fullest.

Success is taking small steps that make a positive impact on my health and the world around me.

Success is managing stress, developing new strength, and becoming more confident in my ability to care for my body and mind.

Success is freeing up all the headspace that used to be full of rules, diets, guilt, and shame—and using it to pursue my passions, make a positive impact on the world around me, and care for the people I love.

Redefining what it means to be successful on your journey to health and wellness is critical to breaking old habits and making lasting changes that support your wellness—in both body and mind.

Reframe #4: Progress Is Worth Celebrating, No Matter How Small

When we think about our health, it's tempting to set big goals or lofty resolutions: *I'm going to lose twenty pounds this year! I'm going to get back into my prepregnancy jeans! I'm going to be swimsuit ready before I go on vacation!* There's nothing wrong with big goals, but setting realistic, attainable goals is proven to increase the likelihood of success. When we attain a goal (even if it's small), we feel accomplished and more confident in our ability to make meaningful changes. This helps us to continue moving forward.

And if we really want to establish new habits and make forward progress, it's not just about the goals; it's also about celebrating our progress along the way. This may sound trivial or unnecessary, but research by B. J. Fogg from the Behavior Design Lab at Stanford University shows that taking time to celebrate small wins helps us to build new habits and attain better results.[4]

The more we shift our focus to what's going well and celebrate progress (no matter how small), the more motivated we are to keep moving forward. Some weeks that will mean celebrating big accomplishments, such as completing a 5K or going for a long hike without feeling fatigued. Other times progress may be as simple as listening to our bodies and drinking a glass of water before filling up a third cup of coffee, or going to bed ten minutes earlier when we're feeling run down. When we intentionally look for and celebrate progress, we will not only realize that

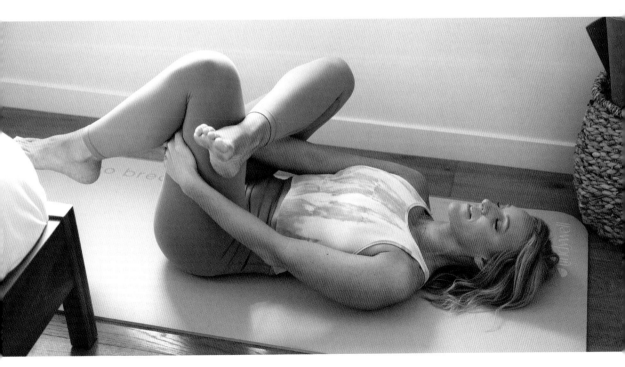

we're doing a better job than we think, we'll also be encouraged and inspired to press on.

For this reason, I promote the fifteen-minute approach to exercise. Most days I aim to do a fifteen-minute workout—that's it! When the goal is small and realistic, it's easier for me to actually do it. (We can all find fifteen minutes, right?) As a result, I'm able to stay consistent with my workouts and feel successful the majority of the time, which spurs me forward on my journey. Instead of feeling like I'll never measure up or I don't have time to exercise, I feel capable and empowered to choose an active lifestyle in the long term.

The same is true for the foods we eat. Making the small shift to start the day with a nourishing breakfast (as opposed to overhauling our entire way of eating) gives us something to celebrate. We can acknowledge the positive habit we're building and allow ourselves to feel successful in our efforts instead of thinking of all the other things we "should" be doing. There's a snowball effect to this: as we experience success in one area, we're inspired to make the next change, one step at a time.

This positive cycle of making small changes and celebrating progress, no matter how small, will spur you onward and help you become more consistent and make greater gains over time.

Reframe #5: It's Possible to Replace Guilt with Grace

It's a natural human tendency to focus more on what's going wrong than on what's going right.[5] If you're like me, you may even believe that if you're hard on yourself or ruminate on what needs to change, it will motivate you to meet your goals. However, I've found through my own experience, through working closely with women around the globe, and through digging into the research that the opposite is true.

Dwelling on failure and daily self-loathing is not an effective recipe for change; in fact, it's more likely to keep us stuck. The approach I've developed is based on embracing a grace-over-guilt mentality. This is a game changer when it comes to repairing your relationship with exercise, food, health, and your body as a whole.

The next time you skip a workout or make a choice that doesn't align with your goals, remember where your worth comes from, and choose grace over guilt. Choose to extend kindness to yourself, acknowledging that it's a normal part of life to have an off day, and take a break from pushing for progress. You're not a failure; you're a human!

When things don't go as planned or when you make a choice that's not in line with your values, it's easy to get trapped in feelings of guilt that lead to a spiral of negative self-talk. These feelings of guilt, shame, and disgust don't spur us on to make better choices in the future; they only keep us stuck. Shame is a terrible motivator for long-term transformation. As Brené Brown puts it, "Shame corrodes the very part of us that believes we are capable of change."[6]

When you're unhappy with a decision you've made, the best thing you can do is to choose grace over guilt and then move forward. Being kind to yourself isn't letting yourself off the hook; it actually helps you make progress in your journey toward health.

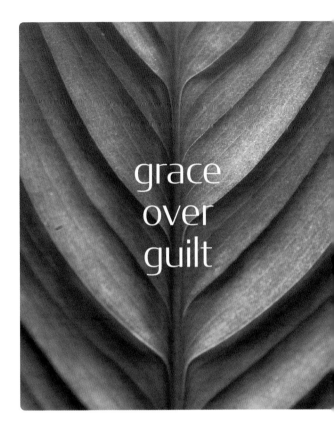

grace over guilt

Give Your Self-Talk a Tune-Up

When it comes to taking care of bodies, the process actually starts in our minds. Researchers from Queen's University in Canada found that people have more than six thousand thoughts per day.[7] The internal conversations we have with ourselves impact how we feel and the choices we make.

Our thoughts affect our self-esteem, our well-being, and our ability to bring about desired changes. If our self-talk is negative, we set ourselves up for an ongoing cycle of trying to implement changes and inevitably falling back into old patterns. But many diet and exercise programs neglect to address the mental aspect of health, which makes it nearly impossible to make changes that last.

As you embark on this journey toward a more balanced, realistic, and sustainable approach to healthy living, it's critical to become aware of the internal conversations that are taking place in your head and shift your thought life toward a more positive, compassionate dialogue. This may sound daunting, especially if you've had an internal voice of criticism for years, but it doesn't have to be overwhelming. Simple changes can have a profound impact.

My inner dialogue used to include a steady stream of negativity. When I was getting dressed and trying to wriggle my jeans over my hips and thighs, I'd beat myself up for not working out more. When I'd order takeout for the third night in a row instead of using the veggies I bought at the grocery store, I'd beat myself up for wasting money and not being able to get it together. When I'd commit to having dessert only on the weekends, I'd beat myself up for my lack of self-control as I pulled the cookies out of the pantry on Monday evening. As a result, I felt like a failure, like I never measured up.

I've come to realize that while negative thoughts may never disappear completely, I can change the conversation that takes place inside my head. I don't have

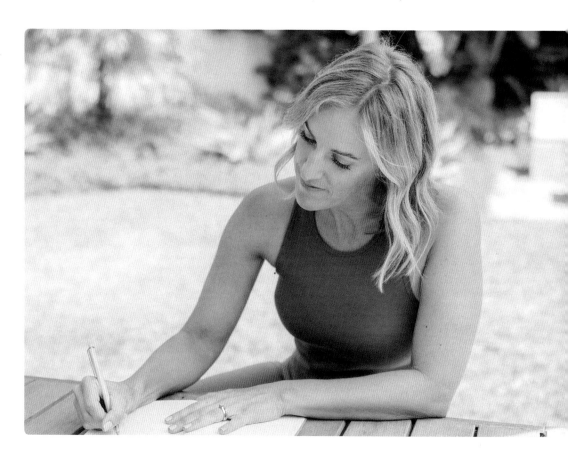

Rest and self-care are so important.
When you take time to replenish your spirit,
it allows you to serve others from the overflow.
You cannot serve from an empty vessel.

Eleanor Brownn

to be ruled by the negative thoughts that have taken up so much of my energy and headspace over the years. When I become aware of the inner dialogue playing out in my mind, I can shift my thoughts to be more productive and more compassionate. You can too.

The first step to improving your inner dialogue is simply to become aware of it. When you find yourself feeling frustrated, discouraged, or overwhelmed, take a moment to breathe and become aware of what you're thinking. Watch your thoughts as a neutral observer. Do these thoughts support your vision for how you want to feel and the person you want to become?

Get curious about your thoughts, without judgment. Begin to notice the way you talk to yourself and how this might affect the way you feel. When that voice in your head isn't as kind as it could be, ask yourself these questions:

- What triggered this thought?

- Does my environment contribute to this thought?

- Where did I learn to speak to myself this way?

- How would I respond to these thoughts if a friend or a loved one were talking to themselves this way?

As you become aware of your thoughts, take some time to journal about them and reflect on the questions above. The simple act of putting your thoughts on paper can help to shift your mindset. While this practice may not feel natural right away, know that it will become more natural the more you do it.

Dr. Kristin Neff, author of *Self-Compassion: Stop Beating Yourself Up and Leave Insecurity Behind*, suggests extending the same compassion to ourselves that we show to others.[8] Think about what you might say to someone you love who is having a bad day or is frustrated over not being able to make progress in an area of their life. Talk to yourself like you would talk to that person.

Rather than thinking, *I missed another workout—I'm such a failure!* try flipping this thought to extend more compassion to yourself. You might say something like "I make time to care for myself and move my body regularly. It's okay if I miss a workout here and there. It's all part of the journey." Even if you're not feeling super positive, you can still extend kindness to yourself by replacing negative thoughts with this simple phrase: "I'm doing the best I can in this moment."

You are worthy of care and kindness, regardless of what you do, what you look like, what you achieve, or how you perform. When I feel negative self-talk surfacing, I remind myself that I am worthy, valuable, and loved by God regardless of the size of my body, the way I perform, or the success I do or do not achieve. When I recognize this truth, everything else falls into place.

The same is true for you, too. You have worth and value simply for being you. You are beautiful, strong, gifted, and worthy just as you are, right now, in this moment. Your worth is inherent. When you embrace this truth, it's easier to extend kindness and grace to yourself, even when your day doesn't go the way you want it to or when you make choices that don't align with your goals.

When we can recalibrate our internal dialogue to speak words of truth to ourselves, we'll eventually begin to understand the fullness of our worth. We'll make more progress, and life will be a lot more enjoyable along the way.

Your Journey Is for You and You Alone

When teaching Pilates classes, I start each routine with a few deep breaths and an opportunity to transition into our time on the mat. This offers a moment to become centered and to tune in to our bodies. Not only does this help us step out of the constant go-go-go and the hurried pace of life, but it also allows us to see what we need that day and set an intention for our time on the mat. That way, no matter what series of exercises I am leading the group through, each person can focus on what they need and how they want to feel when they're done.

When you're doing Pilates, your time on the mat is for you and you alone. The same is true when it comes to your entire wellness journey. I have a hunch you are reading this because you want to live a healthy, balanced, and positive life. You want to feel good, overflow with energy, and enjoy all that life has to offer. You want to be well.

As women, it's easy to consider our needs as secondary to the needs of those around us. We're quick to care for others while hoping we'll have a little time left to take care of ourselves once everyone else's needs are met. But the truth is, your well-being is a priority. Your needs are just as important as everyone else's.

You may be nodding your head in agreement and already living this out, or you may be thinking this sounds good in theory but your day-to-day life doesn't reflect this truth. Or perhaps you're in a situation where you don't have the support you need to care for your basic needs.

> Your needs are just as important
> as everyone else's.

There are often real, significant challenges that stand in the way of being able to prioritize our health and well-being, but together we can make progress. We don't have to neglect the people we love most, and we don't have to overhaul our entire lives. When we decide to prioritize ourselves and care for ourselves in ways that are realistic and sustainable, there will be positive ripple effects—on our own lives and on the lives around us. Maybe your children will benefit from a calmer, more patient parent. Or maybe your grandchild will benefit from a more energetic, pain-free grandparent. Or maybe your colleagues will benefit from a more focused, creative, positive coworker.

Wherever you are on your journey to wellness, I am here to tell you that you are worth it. Your health and well-being are worth prioritizing—for you and you alone. Of course, when you're healthy to your core, other people will benefit too. But as someone created with inherent value, you are reason enough to make your well-being a priority.

[] Put It into Practice

- **Take a few deep breaths,** and reflect on your health in this season of your life. How do you hope to feel as a result of embarking on this journey and embracing a new approach? Take another deep breath, and acknowledge that you are worth the time, energy, and care it takes to feel good and be well.

- **Begin to notice your internal dialogue** throughout the day. Do you speak to yourself kindly, or are you hard on yourself? When you find yourself thinking negatively, try responding with self-compassion by replacing the negative thought with *I'm doing the best I can.*

- **Notice the progress** you're making on your wellness journey, and celebrate that progress, no matter how small! Did you fill a glass of water instead of another cup of coffee? Celebrate that! Did you go for a ten-minute walk instead of sitting in your car waiting for your lunch break to end? Acknowledge that win! Did you make a meal instead of grabbing takeout? Give yourself credit for that effort!

- **Begin to break free** of the all-or-nothing mentality by reminding yourself that every little bit counts and that small changes add up.

- **Make a list** with two columns. In the left column, list the ways you've defined success on your health and wellness journey thus far. In the right column, list deeper ways you can define success.

- **Next time you skip a workout** or make a choice that doesn't align with your goals, choose grace over guilt and keep moving forward.

- **Place a sticky note** on your mirror that says "I'm worth it" to remind yourself that you're worth prioritizing. Your needs matter just as much as those of the people around you, and your self-care is important.

From the Lindywell Community
Shire K.

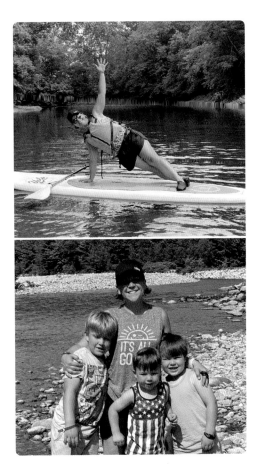

I'm a mom of three little boys, and I ran my own video production company for ten years before switching to a freelance career to spend more time with my boys. My husband recently experienced a heart attack and had open-heart surgery, and that gave us a new outlook on life. Now we're committed to taking better care of ourselves—and we're enjoying life more, as well.

One of the biggest roadblocks I used to face in my health and wellness journey was simply getting started. I would say to myself, *Why not go work out now?* but I'd end up skipping it and scrolling through email instead. I used to feel guilty when I missed a workout for any reason. But shifting my mindset to embrace grace has helped me to overcome this guilt. I know it's okay to take a day off, because sometimes our schedules are too full or we're mentally exhausted. Tomorrow is always a fresh start. When I extend this grace to myself, I'm more likely to look forward to a workout the next day.

I've also come to embrace short workouts. If I'm feeling rushed, I decide to work out for just ten minutes. Once I begin, it feels so good that I usually end up staying on my mat for at least half an hour.

The daily grind of getting the boys ready for school, working, cooking meals, and cleaning up can be exhausting, but when I make time for Pilates, stretching, and self-care, my day is so much better.

Taking the time to move my body gives me energy. I feel stronger, and I'm a better wife, mom, daughter, and friend.

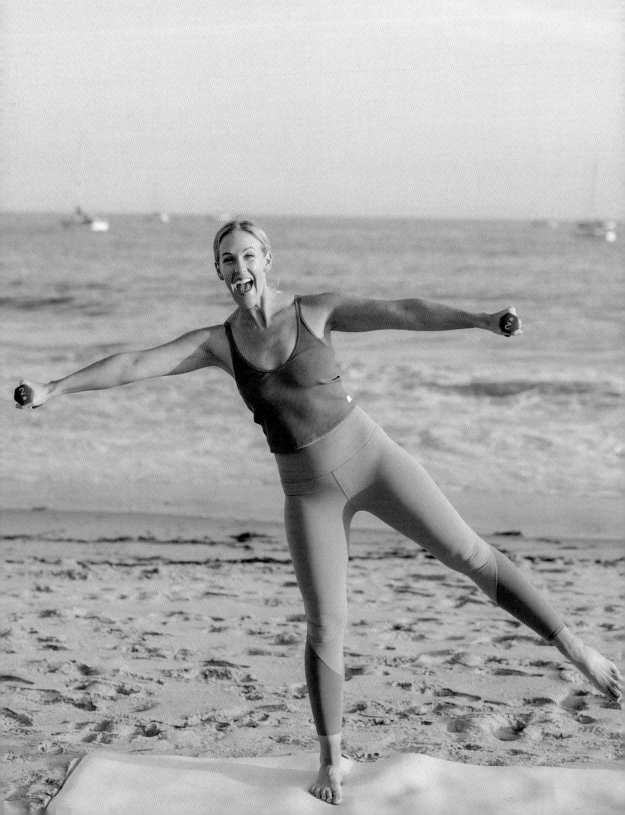

move

Change happens
through movement
and movement heals.

Joseph Pilates

When I was in high school, my girlfriends and I would meet up at the neighborhood rec center to work out. While we were running laps around the track or walking on the treadmill (or checking out cute boys), we'd talk about how many calories we were burning and how we needed to start working out more to get ready for upcoming events like homecoming, prom, or summer vacation.

To this day, I cringe when I think about the elliptical machine. I logged so many hours on that thing in an effort to burn off my last meal or to earn my next one. I wish I could say that mind-set ended in high school, but I lived this

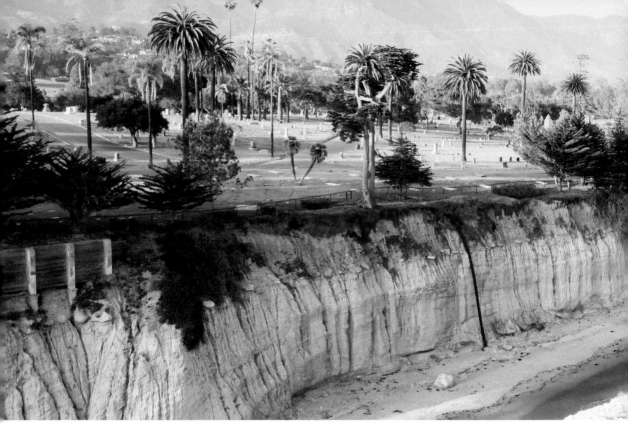

way well into my adult years. Exercise was a box to check purely for the purpose of changing my outward appearance. It had nothing to do with how it made me feel, what it did for my mood, or the actual state of my health.

I'd watch the calorie counter ticking away, wondering why it took so long to burn those darn things. I'd watch the clock (time never moves as slowly as it does on an elliptical machine) and hope there would be a visible change in the size of my thighs by the time I was done.

But don't be fooled—I wasn't a fitness fanatic. Most days I was just trying to muster up the energy to exercise, and I felt uninspired about the process. I went through years of struggle and frustration before I examined my relationship with exercise to determine whether what I was doing was really working for me. I was just doing what I thought I was supposed to do, and I never paused to consider if there was a different—or better—way.

In my twenties, I was working in a high-stress job and started to experience mysterious health symptoms, along with unexplained aches and pains. My neck and back were constantly sore; I had daily stomachaches and was struggling with

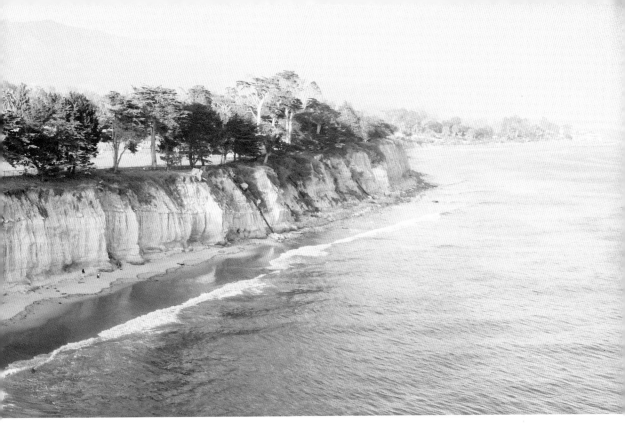

symptoms of anxiety for the first time in my life. I'd always wanted to try Pilates, and I figured it was time to give it a try to ease some of my pain.

I still vividly remember my first class. By the time I left the studio that day, I noticed a shift in the way I felt. Though it was subtle, it was enough to keep me coming back for more.

Pilates provided an entirely new way for me to approach exercise and a tangible way to connect with my body. For the first time, exercise wasn't centered on the number of calories I burned or my outward appearance. I started to understand that the pursuit of health and wellness was about so much more than the size of my jeans, the visibility of cellulite, or the number on the scale.

The impact was so profound that I eventually went on to get my certification as a Pilates instructor. As I continued my journey toward restoring my relationship with my body, food, and exercise, I began to support my clients on their journeys too.

From the beginning of my career, I set out to care for my clients holistically instead of following the typical patterns of the fitness and weight-loss industry. I knew there were women out there who were not being served by the health and fitness industry, because I was one of them. My clients would come to me looking to lose weight before an upcoming vacation or to trim down their arms before their wedding. I listened and acknowledged their goals, and then I encouraged them to look deeper.

I not only provided them with workouts that fit their goals, I also led them on a journey of discovering their true strength and extending themselves more kindness, compassion, and care.

Can losing a few pounds make you feel healthier and proud of your efforts? Sure. Can developing new muscles improve your confidence? Absolutely! But at the end of the day, goals related solely to outward appearance barely scratch the surface of what it means to be well and to live life to the fullest.

If you have a complicated relationship with exercise, take a moment to reflect on a few questions:

- What if exercise doesn't have to feel like a chore?
- What if calorie burn isn't the ultimate goal of moving your body?
- What if more isn't always better?

Exercise doesn't have to be as exhausting or time consuming as we've been led to believe. And here's the really good news: there is gain without pain! Improving your physical health and making exercise a habit can be simple—so simple that it might sound too good to be true. But I promise you, it's not complicated.

Rediscovering the Joy in Movement

It took me years to realize that finding joy in movement is one of the secrets to long-term success. When I started exploring forms of exercise that I genuinely enjoyed and that left me feeling better than when I started, my view of exercise changed. While exercise had once been something I forced myself to do, it became an integral part of my day that I was willing to carve out time for.

During my first Pilates class, I felt the tension melt away from my body in a way I'd never experienced before. I felt present as I listened to the instructor's cues, and I was surprised how quickly the time flew by. Instead of staring at the clock the way I usually did during workouts, I was shocked when the instructor led us into the

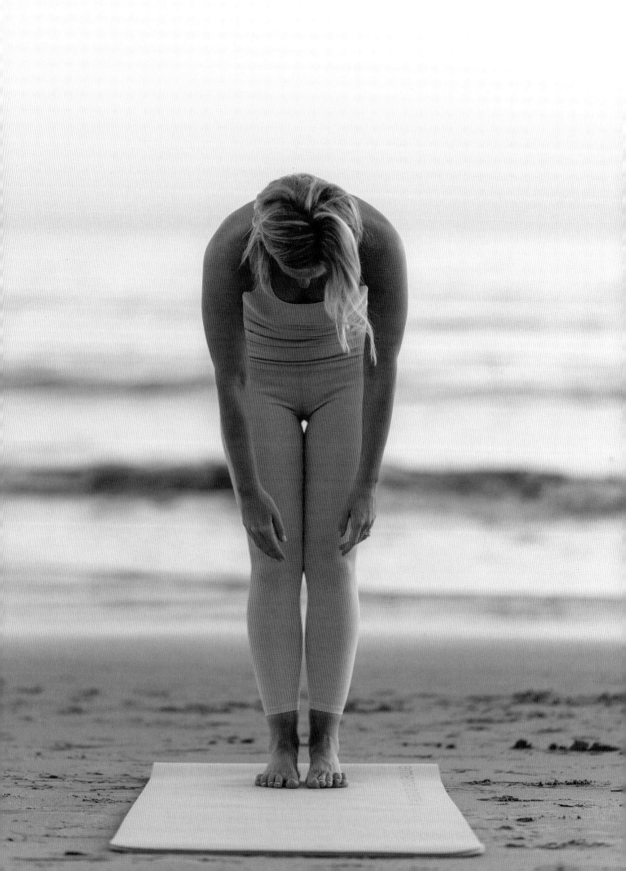

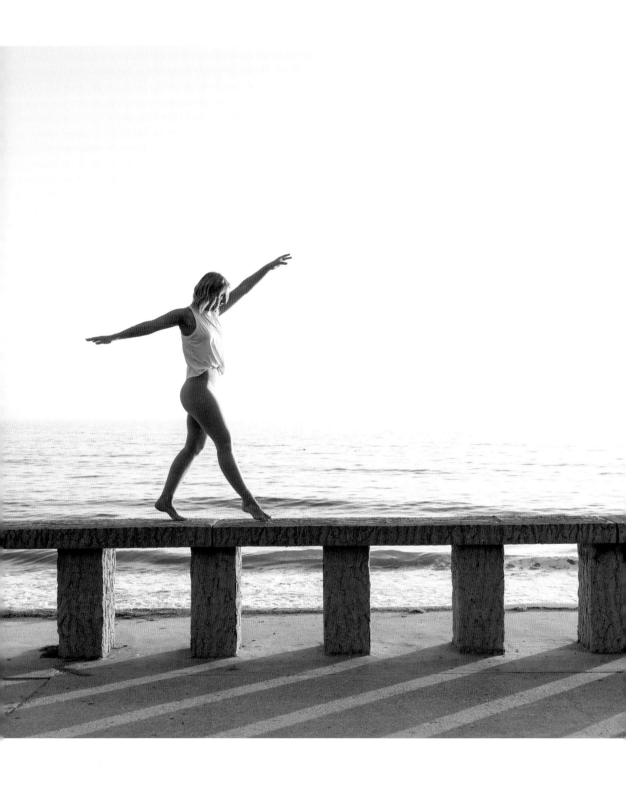

cooldown and wrapped up the class. I remember thinking, *How could we possibly be done already? We just got started!*

When you truly enjoy something and find an activity that engages your mind just as much as it engages your body, you no longer focus on counting the minutes.

I've dedicated more than a decade of my life and career to teaching Pilates and sharing this method of exercise with as many people as possible because it has made such a profound impact on my life, my body, and my relationship with exercise. For you, the activity that brings you joy and freedom might be hiking, swimming, dance class, or morning walks with a friend. Rediscovering what you love and how you genuinely enjoy movement can radically change your relationship with exercise.

In order to discover the kind of movement that sparks joy for you, ask yourself these questions:

- What forms of exercise have I forced myself to do even though they left me feeling worse?
- What beliefs lead me to choose a form of movement I don't enjoy?
- What forms of movement feel more like fun and less like a chore?

Once you've identified types of movement you enjoy, experiment with adding them into your routine in small, realistic ways. Love dancing? Make it a goal to do daily ten-minute dance breaks. Love walking? Add a weekly walk to your routine. Love Pilates? I've got you covered, so just roll out your mat and press play (see the end of this chapter for a free workout).[1] Once you begin to pursue movement you enjoy, you'll notice how much easier it becomes to stay consistent over time.

The Power of Mind-Body Movement

While many forms of movement can help you build strength and feel good, mind-body exercise is a powerful form of movement that benefits everyone, no matter their fitness routine. Mind-body exercise (such as Pilates, yoga, or tai chi) combines mindful movement, controlled breathing, and mental focus to improve strength, mobility, coordination, and control, while also calming the mind and improving mental clarity.

Learning to Listen to Your Body

When starting a new exercise routine, it's normal for your body to feel the effects of new movement patterns—often through sore muscles. Getting in touch with your body will help you determine if the sensation you're experiencing is simply muscle soreness (which typically resolves within a few days) or an injury from overdoing it. Listen carefully to your body, and if you have concerns due to pain or discomfort that persists, reach out to a medical professional.

Mind-body exercise has been shown to lower blood pressure, reduce cortisol levels, and increase levels of dopamine (aka the feel-good hormone). Studies have shown that people who incorporate mind-body exercise into their regular routine have less stress and lower rates of depression. They also cope better with life's challenges and report more feelings of overall satisfaction. Participating in mind-body forms of exercise keeps the brain sharp, improves concentration and focus, and reduces symptoms of anxiety and depression.[2] Put simply, connecting to your body allows you to work with your body, not against it. (More on this in chapter 6.)

Unlike some other forms of mind-body exercise, Pilates does not stem from a religion or a set of spiritual beliefs. While yoga and Pilates may look similar at first glance and may be practiced in similar locations, the exercises are quite different. Pilates is not rooted in a spiritual practice; rather, it was created purely as a system of exercises designed for physical health and conditioning. Pilates implements exercises that are typically performed in repetitions of eight to ten that challenge the body as a whole, with an extra focus on core strength, alignment, and optimal mechanics of movement. In Pilates, you strengthen the connection between your mind and your body, developing an awareness of how your body feels. That means that in addition to the physical benefits, you also reap mental health benefits (such as reduced stress and improved focus).

In Pilates, we focus on form, alignment, and breath. This functional, well-rounded, full-body form of exercise is not only efficient and effective, but it can also be done for a lifetime. The movements are low impact, restorative, and gentle on the joints, yet extremely effective at building muscle, developing strength, reducing pain, increasing bone density, and improving overall mobility. There's a reason Pilates has stood the test of time, through generations and populations. This form of exercise can change your body, and as a result, it can change your life.

Pilates was created by Joseph Pilates in the 1920s. After enduring a number of illnesses as a child, he became motivated to find ways to improve his health through movement. He combined his experiences of training as a boxer, practicing yoga, rehabilitating injured soldiers, and coaching professional dancers with his wife, Clara, to develop an approach to fitness and movement that was originally called *contrology*.

Joseph Pilates was way ahead of his time. He was passionate about counteracting the habits of modern life that negatively impact people's health and well-being, such as poor posture, too much sitting, shallow breathing, and disconnection from nature—all factors that have intensified in the decades since.

Pilates is unique in that it can benefit all people, in all seasons of life. From young to old, from professional athletes to those with fragile bodies, individuals of every age and every body type can adapt the Pilates method to fit their needs. Pilates can be taught and practiced in a studio with state-of-the-art equipment, but it can also be taught and practiced on the mat, with no equipment at all. Both methods are beneficial and effective ways to build strength, restore alignment to the body, prevent injury, refresh the mind, and improve overall focus, coordination, and control.

> Pilates is unique in that it can benefit
> all people, in all seasons of life.

For me, Pilates ignited a new connection between my mind and my body that wasn't about how my body looked but how it felt . . . how *I* felt. It created a new line of communication between my mind and my body that wasn't about burning calories or changing my appearance. Instead, it was about becoming aware of and connecting with my body in a way that was positive, meaningful, and ultimately healing.

If you've spent years of your life dissatisfied with your body or treating it as something that needs to be fixed or changed, there's a good chance there's a disconnection between you and your body. This disconnection is extremely common in our society, especially for women, and it's one of the most common barriers to making positive changes in our health. For many years I saw my body as a problem—something to fix, a point of frustration, a limitation to my happiness. My body was an "other," and I was constantly at battle between my body and myself.

When you've been disconnected from your body for a long time, it's hard to know what connection even feels like. Mind-body exercise such as Pilates provides a practical, approachable way to restore the connection between your mind and your body, and to repair your relationship with exercise. Pilates teaches you to listen to your body and honor its needs, as opposed to pushing through the pain at all costs. When you incorporate Pilates into your routine, you not only strengthen your body and improve your physical health but also care for your mind and improve your mental and emotional well-being.

I wish I had known from a young age what I know now about the connection between the body and the mind. If I had understood that my body was more than a physical representation of my value or a project to constantly be working on, I would have avoided a lot of angst. If I had known how much stress can affect me physically or how much my thoughts impact my well-being, I wouldn't have spent so many years feeling frustrated and discouraged. If I had known that my body wasn't my enemy, I would have been so much happier.

As a mom, I'm dedicated to helping my kids be in tune with their bodies through playing, being mindful, pursuing joy in movement, and watching me model a mind-body approach. Studies show that children and young people who were able to learn to strengthen this mind-body connection had reduced anxiety, increased focus, improved self-image, and fewer behavioral issues.[3]

How Do You Want to Feel?

Given the fact that I run a health and wellness company, I often field a variety of questions from friends and family. One time I was lying by the pool with a friend, watching our kids play a marathon game of Marco Polo, and out of the blue she asked if I knew of any exercises that would make her ankles smaller—particularly the back part. She always noticed women in heels with slim ankles, and hers always felt big in comparison.

PILATES AND THE CORE:

Pilates is known for the way it develops deep core strength. It's recommended for professional athletes, physical therapy patients, and everyone in between. All Pilates exercises strengthen the muscles that make up the core, which includes all the muscles surrounding the trunk: the ab muscles, as well as the diaphragm, the pelvic floor, and the back extensors. During a Pilates workout, you work from the core and stay connected to your center throughout every movement. Other forms of exercise may throw in crunches here and there or focus on sit-ups as the way to get a defined "six-pack," but the truth is, those types of exercises primarily work superficial muscles (literally and figuratively) that don't equate to true core strength. Pilates helps you develop a strong core physically while also helping you connect to the core of who you are and discover your inner strength.

▶▶

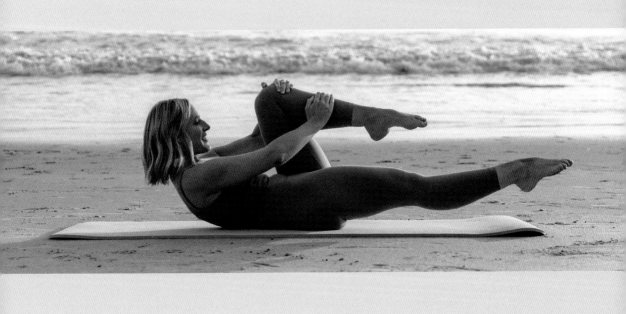

PILATES AND THE SPINE:

Joseph Pilates was known for saying, "If your spine is inflexibly stiff at 30, you are old; if it is completely flexible at 60, you are young."[4] The health of your spine has a significant impact on the way you feel each day and the way you move through the world. As you build a strong core, restore good posture and alignment, and move in a way that supports a healthy spine, your body remains young. It's the ultimate antiaging hack—not in a way that devalues the beauty of age and the wisdom that comes with it but in a way that helps you to maintain an active lifestyle and live life to the fullest through all seasons. The exercises in Pilates also have the potential to make you taller! It's not uncommon for clients to measure an inch taller at their next doctor appointment simply as a result of adding Pilates into their regular routine. Pilates workouts provide benefits not only for your spine but also for stepping into your day, standing tall with confidence.

PILATES AND OPPOSITION:

Another unique element of Pilates workouts is the concept of opposition—working certain muscles while extending other muscles in another direction. For example, as you're reaching your legs one way, you may draw your abdominal muscles the opposite way. As you reach your arms forward, a part of your spine may be reaching backward. Opposition allows you to get the most out of each exercise as you create resistance within your own body, developing strength while also creating length. This unique Pilates principle reminds you that as you embrace opposition in the rest of your life, it can also make you stronger.

PILATES AND FLEXIBILITY:

Strength without flexibility leads to stiffness, rigidity, and pain. Flexibility without strength leads to injury and instability. Pilates helps to improve mobility and range of motion while also building strength, utilizing your own body weight in a low-impact yet highly effective way. When pursuing an exercise routine, it's easy to forget that flexibility matters. Staying mobile allows our bodies to move and adapt without pain or injury, and it's central to staying active and feeling good. As you develop flexibility in your body, you'll notice the many ways this gift of flexibility and resilience can help you weather the stresses of daily life as well.

PILATES AND BALANCE:

Pilates exercises restore balance to the body and incorporate movements that challenge strength and stability. Working through the challenge to remain steady when you feel unstable increases your strength. You may be surprised to discover that balance isn't about staying still; it actually requires the body to constantly adjust, adapt, and respond.

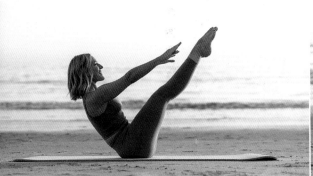
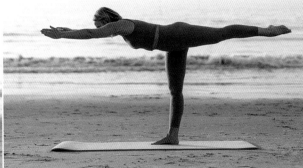

The same is true in daily life. Finding balance isn't a destination; it's a process of listening, adapting, adjusting, and staying focused on what matters most.

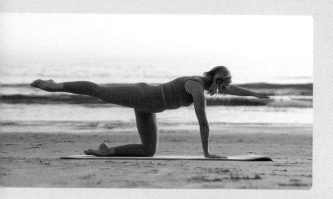

PILATES AND CONTROL:
Joseph Pilates believed that the Pilates method "teaches you to be in control of your body, not at its mercy."[5] The exercises require complete coordination of body and mind, which leads to a unique kind of muscular control. When you feel in control of your movements and your body, it has a ripple effect far beyond your time on the mat. The confidence you uncover as you learn to control the muscles in your body provides a powerful foundation (both mentally and physically) to support you through the ups and downs of life.

PILATES AND ALIGNMENT:
Many forms of exercise focus on power and strength while disregarding the position of the body. Pilates, however, teaches you to become aware of your alignment as you move, being mindful of whether your head is in line with your spine, your shoulders are over your hips, or your rib cage is square to the mat. While these adjustments may be small, the impact is significant. Working in proper alignment maximizes the efficiency and effectiveness of each exercise. As you note the alignment in your body, you may notice that the same is true in your life. When you're out of sync with your values and priorities, your day-to-day responsibilities feel hard and slow. But when you're aligned, everything flows.

I smiled and told her, as someone who inherited what we have lovingly dubbed the "Long family cankles," I'm not the one to ask. I also told her that slimming ankles is not my area of expertise. Instead, my work is to remind people that they don't need to worry about the size of their ankles to begin with.

Another friend recently asked me what workout she can do to fix her "jiggly arms" (her words, not mine). While I know plenty of exercises that will target those muscles in her arms, my first inclination was to ask questions to help her dig a little deeper.

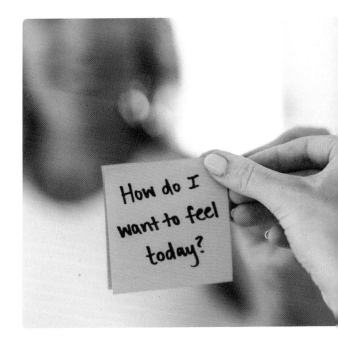

- Why are 'jiggly arms' a bad thing?

- Is this situation interfering with your ability to live the life you want to live?

- Does it make it hard for you to get through the day?

These types of questions are worth exploring. Sometimes we spend years thinking about how we need to "fix" our bodies through exercise when they may not need fixing at all.

Shifting the focus from what you want to fix to how you want to feel is one of the most important and effective changes you can make when it comes to moving your body. As exercise becomes a tool to help you feel a certain way (unrelated to how you look), it brings a refreshing sense of freedom.

What if you don't have to stress about the size of your thighs or the tone of your arms in order to be well? What if you could become clear on how you want to feel and experience a strong internal motivation to do what will help you feel that way?

Consider asking yourself each morning, *How do I want to feel today?* and then take the actions that will support that feeling. Some days you'll want to feel strong and powerful, so you'll choose a workout that leaves you feeling accomplished. Some days you'll want to feel calm, centered, and relaxed, so you'll choose a form of movement that leaves you feeling that way. Some days you'll want to feel more rested, so sleep may take the place of that early-morning alarm. When you focus on how you want to feel rather than on what you want to fix, you'll rediscover the joy in movement, and it will be easier to be consistent in choosing a healthy, active lifestyle.

The Emotional Benefits of Moving Your Body

If you're like me and most women I know, you have a lot on your plate. There are always things we need to think about and items on our never-ending to-do list. Add to that the overwhelming amount of information that's thrown at us from social media, the news, emails, and podcasts, and it's easy to feel overwhelmed. It may seem like exercise is just one more item to add to our list of responsibilities, but in fact, it's something that gives us the reserves we need to navigate all that's on our plate. In such an information-saturated society, we tend to stay solely in our heads and neglect moving our bodies. When we connect with our bodies, it can change the way we feel and function, both physically and mentally.

Did you know that taking time to move also helps us move emotions through our bodies? I used to think this was a little "woo-woo," but I've seen this play out time after time with my clients and in my own life. Over the years I've seen client after client cry unexpectedly during Pilates class. This is therapeutic release—something that can happen when you move through new ranges of motion and release tension from the body. I've seen other clients come into a session feeling completely stressed or overwhelmed and walk out feeling refreshed, energized, and more positive about their lives.

When I started noticing this pattern, it led me on a deep dive into the way we can heal our bodies and change our emotions through movement. It turns out that when we move our bodies, we support the brain's ability to process our emotions in a healthy and effective way.[6] The simple act of moving the body resets the parasympathetic nervous system to take us out of fight-or-flight mode and into a place of calm and clarity.

When you feel overwhelmed and you're not sure what to do, get moving. Lace up your shoes and go for a walk. Roll out your mat and do a few exercises. Turn up the music and dance around the room. Moving our bodies is good not only for our physical health but also for our minds.

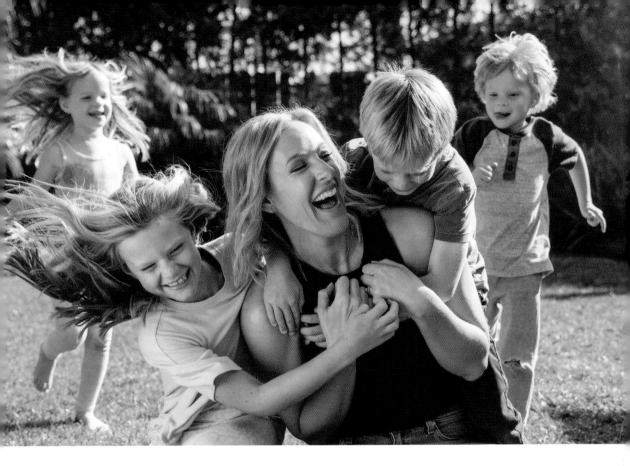

Be Intentional, but Stay Flexible

It's true what they say: "You don't find time for exercise; you *make* time for exercise." But can I confess to you that as a mom of four little ones (who also runs a quickly growing company), I kind of hate that phrase? It's hard for me to make time for exercise in the season I'm in—harder than it's ever been (apart from when I was nursing twins around the clock while also working and chasing toddlers).

As frustrating as this saying is, however, I know it's true. I rarely (if ever) stumble upon free time that lends itself to the perfect opportunity to exercise. If I find a moment of free time, I usually want to collapse onto my bed to hide for a few precious moments of rest and quiet. If you're caring for other people, trying to pay the bills, or keeping your world afloat, you can probably relate. Even if you're in a season where your schedule is less structured, it can still be hard to get moving because there are always other things that need to be done.

To stay consistent with exercise and make positive changes to your health, it's imperative to set clear goals and plan ahead. Having an intentional plan for how and when you'll exercise will help you build it into your weekly routine more than hoping it will happen by chance.

But it's just as important to remain flexible. You might miss your morning work-out because of an unexpected phone call or an interruption by a child or a missed alarm, but if your plan is flexible, the change won't throw you off course for the rest of the day. You can find time to work out later in the afternoon, or if that doesn't work, simply choose grace over guilt and start fresh the next day. (I do this often.) Having a plan but keeping it flexible is one of the best ways to stay consistent, reap the benefits of movement, and experience tangible forward progress.

Consistency over Intensity

If there's one struggle I hear about repeatedly from people, it's the challenge to stay consistent with exercise. I get it—I've struggled with this too. My old pattern went something like this. I'd reach a tipping point (such as gaining weight, feeling lethargic, or wanting to get in shape for an upcoming trip or special event) and decide I needed to get it together once and for all. I'd start a new exercise routine (which also meant getting all the gear, cute workout clothes, and new shoes). With this renewed sense of motivation, I'd start a new routine and stick with it for a few days. But then something would come up—a work deadline, having a friend in town, getting sick, traveling, etc.—and I'd start skipping workouts. Eventually I'd feel so discouraged at my inability to stick with my workout program that I'd throw in the towel altogether. (Remember that all-or-nothing mentality that needs to be reframed?) Since I couldn't keep up with the plan, I'd quit. Then I wouldn't do any-thing for a few weeks or a few months (sometimes longer) until I hit another tipping point. Then I'd start the whole cycle over again—including more new clothes and gear, because for some reason that's always the easiest step to take.

Small changes can lead to big transformations.

Is this pattern familiar to you? If so, you're not alone. I hear from women on a daily basis who are practically paralyzed with discouragement over their exercise spirals. You may be tempted to think the problem is that you're just not motivated enough or disciplined enough. But that isn't actually the issue! The truth is, most workout programs require an unrealistic amount of change and commitment. As a result, they lead to a cycle of starting and stopping, making it nearly impossible to stay consistent and solidify long-term habits.

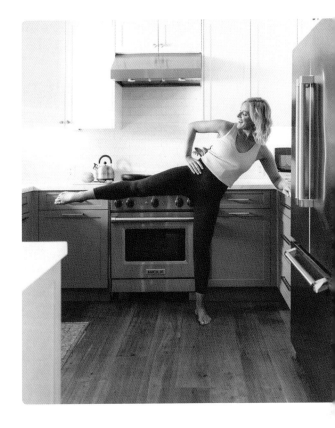

So what can we do? We can start by understanding that we're human and that building a new habit isn't as easy as signing up for a gym membership, buying a piece of fancy equipment, or purchasing a new pair of running shoes. We need to start smaller and shift our focus to pursuing consistency over intensity. It's more important to be intentional day in and day out about moving and taking care of our bodies than to go big for a few days and then do nothing.

I've seen this concept proven in my own life and with women I've taught for more than a decade, but this strategy is also supported by research. Dr. B. J. Fogg, founder of the Behavior Design Lab at Stanford University, sums it up this way: "In order to design successful habits and change your behaviors, you should do three things. Stop judging yourself. Take your aspirations and break them down into tiny behaviors. Embrace mistakes as discoveries and use them to move forward."[7]

Recently I was chatting with a member of our online community who wanted to get in shape and feel better. She decided to start a new diet (removing multiple food groups), work out five times a week, and meditate each morning. While I admired her desire to make positive changes, I've seen other people make the same mistake in biting off more than they could chew. I encouraged her to focus on one small change at first, such as exercising for fifteen minutes at a time, two to three times a week. That's it. She was skeptical, but she agreed.

After a few weeks, she shared that she'd been consistent with her new plan and was actually enjoying the process. It felt good to be successful! Now that she'd developed one small habit that supported her goals, her motivation was high. I encouraged her to add one more small change. She decided to stick with her routine of exercising three times a week and add a goal of cooking dinner at home three nights a week instead of getting takeout. Not only was this approach more realistic and sustainable, it was also more enjoyable.

If you're trying to make changes in your life, focus on the basics and keep it simple. Start by moving your body more often and discovering what forms of movement you genuinely enjoy. This could look like sneaking a few short walks into your day, taking regular stretch breaks while you work, dancing around the living room at the end of a long day, or taking the stairs when you're running errands. The next time you need a break from a project you're working on, consider taking a ten-minute walk instead of scrolling social media. You'll return more refreshed, energized, and focused.

Studies have found that just ten minutes of light to moderate exercise every day of the week results in an 18 percent lower risk of early death, a 12 percent lower risk of dying from cardiovascular issues, and a 14 percent lower risk of dying from cancer.[8] On top of those physical benefits, short bursts of movement get your blood flowing throughout your body, which results in mood boosts, increased energy, and improved focus.

Before you get caught up in complicated workout plans and daunting commitments, shift your focus to moving your body as often as you can, in ways you actually enjoy. Every little bit counts.

Small changes can lead to big transformations. This is the secret to long-term success. This is the ticket to a life of wellness and balance.

Building Your Confidence Muscle

Studies show that with each new diet a person tries, they stick with it for a shorter and shorter amount of time.[9] One possible reason for this is that with each unsuccessful attempt, you lose confidence in yourself. This cycle will continue unless you take a different approach and find a way to build confidence in your ability to make lasting changes.

The key to breaking this loop is to start small. Focus on short bits of movement, interspersed throughout your day, and notice how this makes you feel. Start with one ten-minute movement break in your day, and let that be enough as you get started. Celebrate that ten-minute accomplishment (it's important to celebrate progress, no matter how small!), and then as that habit solidifies, use the same approach to increase your movement by ten more minutes. Remember, this is a lifelong journey. Slow, steady, and realistic wins the race every single time.

As you take small steps and start experiencing success, you'll rebuild your confidence in yourself and your ability to show up for yourself. There will be ripple effects in other areas of your life as well. You may notice that you're able to stick to your word more effectively or that you're able to break large projects down into more achievable steps. Because you've been able to show up for yourself and make progress, you may find yourself taking steps toward the career change you've been wanting to make or taking on new challenges that would have once felt intimidating. When you learn to trust yourself with self-care, you learn to trust yourself, period.

If you already have a solid routine in place and you love what you're doing, take time to celebrate your progress and the confidence you've built. Remind yourself that all movement is good movement and that your worth is not determined by the length or intensity of your workout. Some days you might push it and challenge yourself; other days you might slow it down and move more gently. A balanced life leaves room for both and releases you from the expectation that more is always better or that there can't be gain without pain.

When we recognize the value of exercise—that it's about so much more than logging hours at the gym or attaining a certain number on the scale—and when we find something we truly enjoy, it can change our entire outlook on moving our bodies. And as we experience small victories with exercise, we will build our confidence not just in what our bodies can do but in who we are at the very core of our being.

Put It into Practice

- **Set an alarm** on your phone to alert you three times a day to get up and move your body. It might be a few stretches, a short Pilates workout, or a brisk walk around the block. Or you might just turn on your favorite music and dance. Remember, every little bit counts!

- **Think about your spine** as you go through your day. Create a mental trigger (such as when you're sitting at a stoplight or when your phone rings) to remind you to lengthen your spine toward the sky.

- **Create a plan** of doing ten to fifteen minutes of intentional movement each day. If you aren't sure what to do, set a timer on your phone and dance around the room, or try the simple Pilates workout included at the end of this chapter. It is suitable for all levels!

- **Shift your focus** from what you want to fix to how you want to feel. Start your day by asking yourself how you want to feel, and then make a list of things you can do to help you feel that way.

Simple Pilates Workout

If you've never tried Pilates and aren't sure where to begin, or if you want a workout that will strengthen and stretch your entire body, scan the QR code to access a video of this quick 15-minute Pilates basics workout.

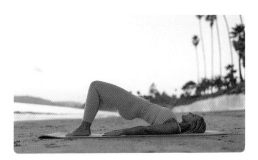
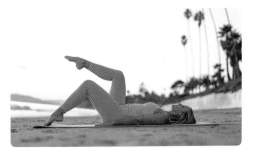

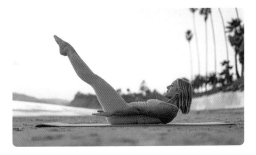
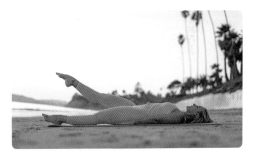

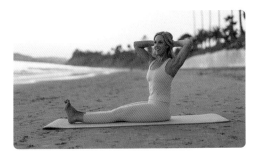

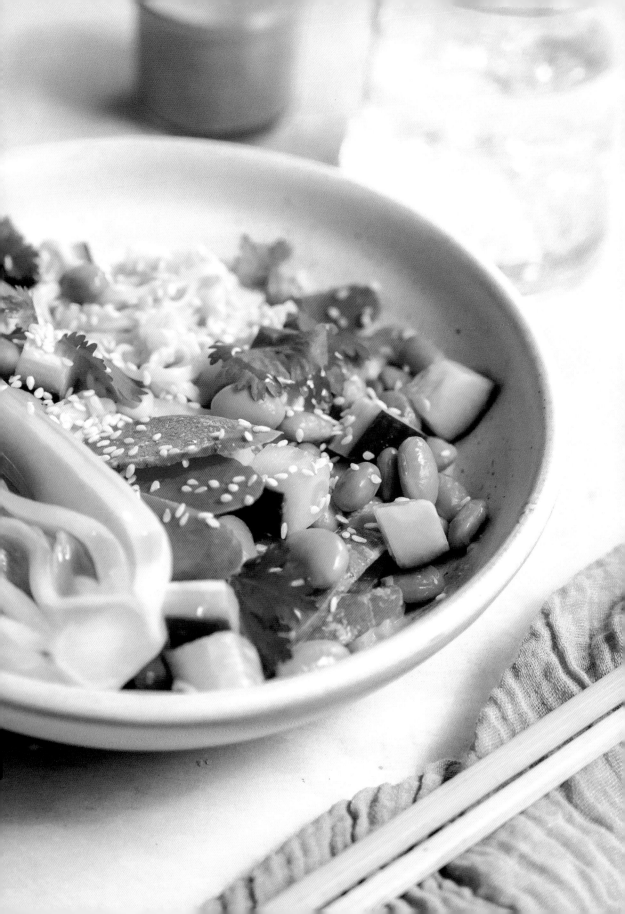

Chapter 3

nourish

Food is not just fuel. Food is about family, food is about community, food is about identity. And we nourish all those things when we eat well.

Michael Pollan

I was fourteen when I overheard my friends talking about the new diet they'd started. We were getting ready for a dance competition, and instead of goofing off or having fun, they were talking about how many points they had left to eat. These were girls I looked up to and admired. They were thin, active, and fit, and they had no good reason to be on a diet.

This was my introduction to dieting. Learning to count calories, restricting my food intake, taking diet pills, feeling guilty about eating food that wasn't "healthy"—this became the norm in my social circle, in the magazines I read, and in the commercials I saw on television.

I grew up in the midst of the diet-culture boom. Food companies had caught on to our quest for thinness, and they marketed their products to solve all our problems. They perpetuated an ideal body shape, recognizing there was big money to be made as we struggled with desiring to change our bodies while also wanting to enjoy one of life's greatest pleasures: food.

My internal struggle continued throughout high school. I was living in constant tension between loving food and thinking I should eat less of it. Since I was a dancer, my body was constantly on display. I spent hours in front of wall-to-wall mirrors wearing spandex leotards and comparing my body to those of the other girls in the room. Fittings for costumes and uniforms put a spotlight on my size and my measurements, inviting all to see—and judge. As a result, food became a source of stress for me.

While your story may differ from mine, I'm willing to bet you've had your own challenges in your relationship with food. Whether you binge in the evenings, eat in secret, restrict yourself before special events, or find yourself just plain confused by what's healthy and what's not these days, you're not alone.

Food is complicated. It's emotional; it's celebratory; it's functional; it's comforting. It's all those things. But it doesn't have to be all consuming. It's possible to approach food in a way that frees up our headspace while supporting good health. In the Lindywell approach, we have a philosophy of embracing freedom and getting rid of guilt. We ditch the strict rules, forgo the shame, release the all-or-nothing mindset, and discover an enjoyable, balanced approach to eating.

From Restriction to Nourishment

To change our relationship with food, we must first change the way we think about it. Food is a gift. Food nourishes our bodies from the inside out. It's miraculous to think how the nutrients in certain foods can reduce our risk for cancer, support muscle growth, improve brain function, and boost immunity. Not only does food affect the physiological processes that happen in our bodies on a day-to-day basis, but it also affects the way we feel. Food can slow the aging process, improve quality of life, and increase health span (the years you can live and enjoy life, free from serious disease).[1] Put another way, food is a gift, designed to nourish and support our bodies in very specific ways.

A significant shift happens when we begin to view food as a source of nourishment instead of a vice we're constantly battling. Our bodies need specific nutrients to be well nourished. We need things like water, minerals, fat, protein, and carbohydrates to function optimally. The simple shift of asking ourselves, *Will this provide my body the nourishment it needs?* instead of *Should I eat this?* will help transform the way we think and the choices we make.

You may be hesitant about making this switch, fearing what it would look like to let go of control around food. If that's where you are, I understand—I used to feel that way too. If you've spent years dieting, it's hard to know whether you can trust yourself to eat in a healthy way without rigid guidelines. However, the research proves that diets simply do not work. Not only do they not work, they can actually hurt.

Dieting wreaks havoc on your hormones and slows your metabolism. Repeatedly losing and regaining weight is linked to strokes, diabetes, cardiovascular disease, and impaired immune function. And that doesn't factor in the harmful impact on your brain, emotional well-being, and confidence. So we have good reason, backed by evidence, to embrace a different approach.[2]

Shifting the Focus Away from the Scale

Knowing what to eat and what not to eat has never been more confusing. What was once recommended is now problematic, and it's only a matter of time before the next health discovery will come onto the scene and change the conversation yet again.

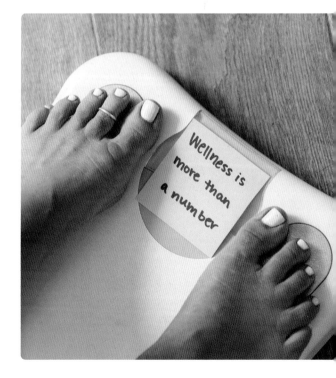

In all my years trying various diets, I became discouraged because what was considered "healthy" kept changing. This led me to find out what is agreed upon to be nourishing to the body as opposed to harmful or problematic to the body. In my search, I discovered that when you fill your diet with foods that support healthy blood-sugar levels, it has an anti-inflammatory effect on the body.

This was a big mental shift for me. I had always thought of foods as "good" or "bad" based simply on calorie count or fat content. When I learned that food affects our physiology in ways far beyond those two metrics, my eyes were opened to the power of food. What I ate could help me balance blood sugar and reduce inflammation—two things at the center of good health *and* healthy weight maintenance. This meant I could eat in a way that would support a healthy weight while also nourishing my body.

This discovery was clarifying in my quest to eat well—and it was refreshing, too. It simplified the decision-making process in a beautiful way. It meant no counting, no tracking, no measuring—just focusing on foods that provide my body with the nourishment it needs to thrive and foods that reduce inflammatory markers that lead to sickness and disease. More than a decade later, this approach continues to be just as valuable and effective in supporting a healthy lifestyle as when I first embraced it.

So what exactly is inflammation? Our bodies all have some level of inflammation at different times. There is helpful inflammation (acute), which is necessary for healing and helps your body when you get an injury or a virus (think redness around a cut as it heals or a fever that heats up the body to kill a virus). Acute inflammation is usually short term, and it's essential to our survival.

Chronic inflammation, on the other hand, is harmful because it can lead to disease or illness if left unchecked. While many factors contribute, some common causes of chronic inflammation include pro-inflammatory foods (see sidebar), chronic stress (emotional or physical), lack of sleep, smoking, and acute inflammation that doesn't resolve on its own. Chronic inflammation can be a sign that something more serious is going on in the body. It is linked to heart disease, Alzheimer's disease, autoimmune diseases, cancer, and diabetes.[3]

The good news is that inflammation is something we have the power to influence through our lifestyle choices. When we reduce stress, move our bodies, and fill our diet with nourishing foods, we can reduce inflammation, which is one of the most important actions we can take for our health. While there are a number of ways to reduce chronic inflammation, being intentional with food is one of the best ways to get started.[4]

If you're wondering if your body is dealing with chronic inflammation, you can

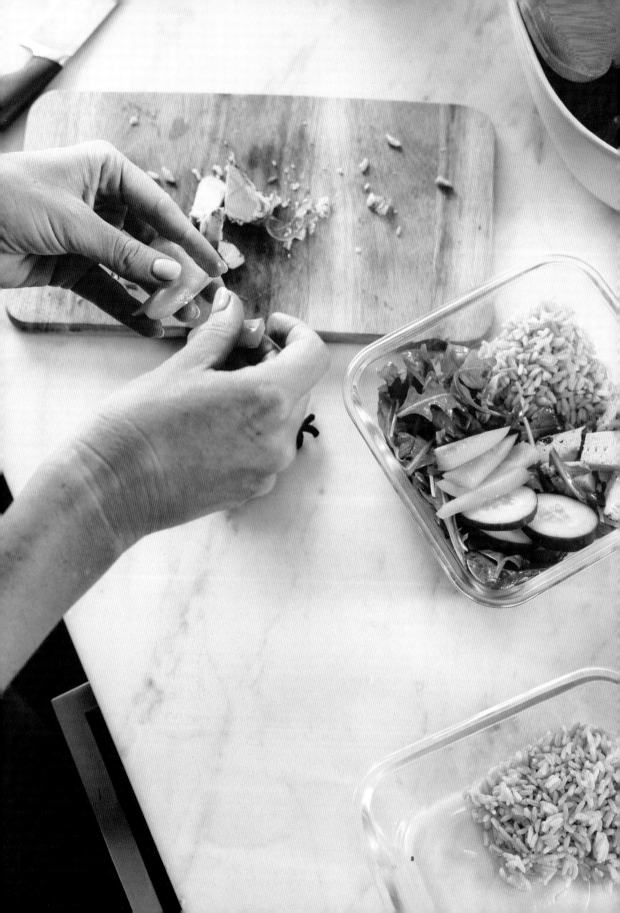

Pro-Inflammatory Foods

The following foods are generally known to increase inflammation:

- sugar
- alcohol
- refined carbohydrates (such as white bread and pastries)
- processed foods (such as chips, crackers, cereal, and other packaged goods)
- fried foods
- processed meats
- dairy and gluten (for some)

Anti-Inflammatory Foods

The following foods are generally known to reduce inflammation:

- berries
- cherries
- turmeric
- green tea
- green leafy vegetables
- cruciferous vegetables
- olive oil
- tomatoes
- fatty fish
- nuts

Signs of Chronic Inflammation in the Body

- body pain
- chronic fatigue and insomnia
- depression, anxiety, and mood disorders
- gastrointestinal complications such as constipation, diarrhea, and acid reflux
- weight gain or weight loss
- frequent infections
- skin rashes
- excessive mucus production

talk to your doctor about assessing your inflammation levels. Here are some of the tests you might request: white blood cell count, sedimentation rate (ESR), and high sensitivity C-reactive protein (hs-CRP).[5] While you're at it, you may want to request a full blood work panel that checks hormone levels as well. If you have specific concerns regarding hormones, you can also request a salivary test that measures hormone levels throughout the day for more comprehensive results.

Practicing Mindfulness around Food

Food is a gift that can nourish and support your body and help you feel your best. It's also a great source of comfort and pleasure—something that's meant to be enjoyed. We all know moderation is key, and while that sounds great in theory, it's hard to put into practice. If you've ever said you're just going to have one cookie and ended up eating far more than that, you know what I mean.

So what can we do? Instead of fighting the constant battle of moderation with sheer willpower, we can utilize the tool of mindfulness.

> Food is a gift that can nourish
> and support your body
> and help you feel your best.

Mindfulness is the practice of maintaining a nonjudgmental state of awareness about your thoughts, emotions, or experiences on a moment-by-moment basis. This may sound daunting, but it's simply about paying attention to the present moment. For me, that looks like asking myself, *Will this food choice provide the nourishment my body truly needs?* It also means listening to my hunger level, noticing what I'm craving, and doing my best to focus on the food I'm eating instead of looking at a screen (this is a work in progress for me).

Before I started applying the concept of mindfulness to my eating habits, I could never figure out when to stop eating. Either I was making decisions based solely on keeping my calorie count low, which left me hungry and longing for my next meal, or I was throwing caution to the wind, which left me walking out of restaurants

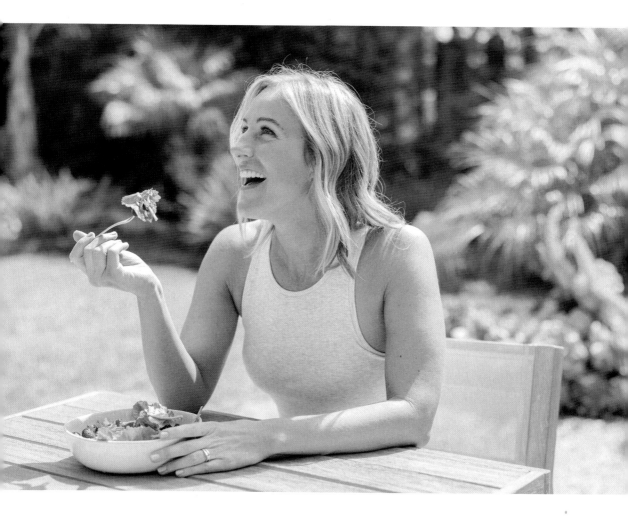

feeling so full I could hardly breathe. I didn't know how to listen to my body's cues (more on this in chapter 4).

Applying the art of mindfulness when we eat helps us recognize when we're acting out of habit rather than truly nourishing our bodies or responding to a need. Eating out of habit can look like an afternoon trip to the vending machine or coffee shop for a sugary pick-me-up or snacking while watching a show at night, regardless of whether we're truly hungry. When we bring mindfulness into our relationship with food, we're able to pause and pay attention instead of making mindless decisions. When our minds have an opportunity to connect with our bodies, our decisions can support the lifestyle we want.

In addition to helping us pay attention to what we truly need, mindfulness helps us slow down, relax, and breathe, which can also improve our digestion and our bodies' ability to absorb the nutrients of the foods we're eating.

While it's tempting to follow a diet that tells you exactly what to eat, how much to eat, and when to eat, becoming mindful about your food choices and mealtimes is more impactful in the long term. As you become intentional about food, you'll begin to notice the way certain foods make you feel. You'll increase your awareness about the quantity of food your body needs. You'll naturally start to gravitate toward foods and choices that support your wellness because you notice that they help you feel your best. You'll break free of old habits that no longer serve you. When choosing to have a dessert, you'll do so with intention and truly enjoy it. Not only will you learn to feed yourself with intention, but you'll also be able to enjoy food as the gift it is. You'll savor flavors, chew more slowly (which helps reduce bloating and improves digestion), breathe more deeply, and feel more satisfied.

> But perfection is not required for progress,
> and we give ourselves grace.

I'm the first to admit that with my busy lifestyle, I don't do this perfectly. There are many nights I find myself practically inhaling my food as children scream for more water or yell for help going to the bathroom. There are days I'm late for work and grab a protein bar as I run out the door, eating it mindlessly while thinking about the many tasks ahead of me. But perfection is not required for progress, and we give ourselves grace. Don't forget that every little bit counts, and small changes add up.

Making Friends with Cravings

Cravings have a bad reputation. They're often thought of as a problem—something we don't want, something we'd prefer to do away with altogether. In reality, there are two layers to cravings: what's happening on an emotional level and what's happening on a physical level.

My cravings were the highest they've ever been during the seasons I restricted the food I was eating. If I told myself I couldn't have sweets, all I wanted was sweets.

If I told myself I couldn't have seconds, all I wanted was another helping. On an emotional level, it's natural to want what we can't have.

Another emotional component to cravings comes into play because we associate certain feelings with food. For example, when you're worried, you may crave foods that bring a feeling of comfort and security. When you're bored, you may crave foods that bring a sense of fun, such as a delectable treat or a fancy cocktail.

On a physiological level, cravings can be a powerful way to tell us what our bodies need. We often want salty foods when we need more sodium; we crave cold beverages when we're hot and dehydrated; we look for sugar when we're short on sleep and need a quick boost of energy. It's amazing the way our bodies can self-regulate. But these feelings can also be unnaturally manufactured or perpetuated by the foods we eat.

When my diet was full of processed diet foods, my cravings were off the charts. Highly processed foods are typically low in fiber and high in sugar, which leads to a blood sugar imbalance. When blood sugar is out of balance, your cravings are likely to increase. Alternatively, when you fuel your body with nutrient-rich, whole (meaning minimally processed or in their most natural form) foods, you'll naturally be eating more fiber, protein, and healthy fats. These nutrients trigger feelings of satisfaction and satiety, and as result, fewer cravings.[6]

Foods that are high in salt, sugar, and fat also trigger the feel-good center, or reward center, of the brain, leading us to reach for foods that give us the good feelings we crave. The food industry has increasingly engineered "hyperpalatable" foods that light up the reward centers in our brains, creating a desire for "more, more, more!" (think chips, cookies, crackers, and candy).

According to the State of Childhood Obesity project, "Food, beverage and restaurant companies spend almost $14 billion per year on advertising, more than 80 percent of which promotes fast food, sugary drinks, candy, and unhealthy snacks." Children are a target audience, and children in communities of color are disproportionately targeted. According to studies, kids and teens see "an average of eleven to twelve ads per day on television for these types of products. . . . African American children and teens see more than twice as many ads for sugary drinks than their white peers."[7]

The challenge is even greater for those who live in "food deserts"—areas with limited access to affordable, healthy food options (especially fresh produce). More than two million people in the United States live over a mile away from a grocery

Balancing Blood Sugar

Blood sugar, also known as glucose, is a necessary energy source for the body. However, it's critical to keep blood sugar balanced. As Jessie Inchauspé explains in *Glucose Revolution*, "Glucose is our body's main source of energy. We get most of it from the food we eat, and it's then carried into our bloodstream to our cells. Its concentration can fluctuate greatly throughout the day, and sharp increases in concentration—I call them *glucose spikes*—affect everything from our mood, our sleep, our weight, and our skin to the health of our immune system, our risk for heart disease, and our chance of conception."[8]

You may have heard of glucose as it relates to diabetes (a result of high glucose levels in the blood), but glucose levels affect all of us and how we feel day to day. When our glucose is out of balance, it often has a domino effect that throws other systems in our body out of balance.

So what can we do? Put simply, we can aim for a combination of protein, healthy fat, and fiber in our meals and snacks. This isn't meant to be another food rule to follow—think of it as a guideline for balancing food in a way that nourishes your body and helps you feel the way you want to feel.

Here are a few examples of meals and snacks that include a balance of these three nutrients:

- **sliced apple** (fiber) and **almond butter** (fat and protein)
- **orange slices** (fiber) and **cashews** (fat and protein)
- **carrot sticks** (fiber) and a **hard-boiled egg** (fat and protein)
- **omelet** (fat and protein) with **sautéed vegetables** (fiber)
- **salmon** (fat and protein) with **roasted vegetables** (fiber)

Understanding how to pair foods to balance glucose can help you maintain your energy level, reduce stress, reduce cravings, and feel your best.

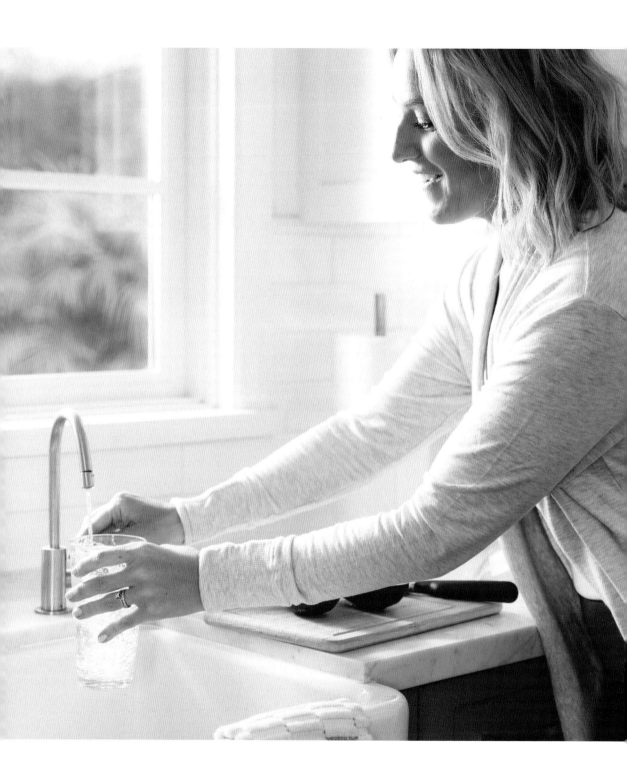

store and don't own a car. Studies have found that wealthy districts have three times as many supermarkets as low-income ones and that white neighborhoods have four times as many supermarkets as areas with predominantly Black residents.[9] This is unconscionable. Food and beverage companies, as well as the stores that sell these products, know how hard it is to resist these "hyperpalatable" foods, and we've been influenced to see them as staples in our diet and our children's diet.

Many other factors can affect our cravings, such as sleep, stress, medications, and hormonal fluctuations. But it's important to know that cravings don't have to be the enemy—they can be helpful in making sure our bodies get what they need.

If it's midafternoon, your energy is waning, and you're craving something sweet, you can honor that craving for more energy with a big glass of water, a handful of nuts, and a sprinkling of dark chocolate chips. This type of snack will give your body the energy it needs while also satisfying the desire for something sweet. In the evening, if you're craving a crunchy, salty snack while watching your favorite show, instead of reaching for a bag of chips, consider apple slices with salted nut butter for dipping. You'll satisfy the craving while providing your body with nourishment to support good health.

As we become mindful of which foods trigger cravings and which foods don't, and as we understand the effect of highly processed foods, we are empowered to respond wisely to these cravings.

Staying Hydrated

Now let's bring it back to the basics. What if I told you there was a simple change that could transform your health, boost your energy, improve your skin, strengthen your immune system, improve digestion, and support your body's natural detoxification process? Sounds a little too good to be true, doesn't it? But it's true, not to mention free and easy to implement. This simple change is drinking more water.

Staying hydrated is perhaps the most underrated habit you can choose for your health. For most of us, clean water is widely accessible. It's something we can easily add to our daily routine without carving out extra time or investing a lot of money.

You've probably heard that up to 60 percent of the human body is made of water. But that percentage increases when we look at essential internal organs such as the brain and the heart (73 percent water), the lungs (83 percent), the skin

(64 percent), and the kidneys (79 percent).[10] Here are just a few of the functions our bodies need water for:

- We need hydration so our cells can absorb the nutrients they need to function effectively.

- We need hydration so our cells can regenerate and reproduce to keep us healthy and strong.

- We need hydration so our bodies can remove toxins (no juice cleanse necessary!).

- We need hydration for the synovial fluid in our joints so we can move freely, without pain or stiffness.

- We need hydration to support the digestive process and ease digestive discomfort.

Despite all these benefits, we often fill up on coffee or soda, with water as an afterthought. The simple habit of drinking more water can improve sleep, focus, memory, and mood. It's a key component in looking and feeling young. Even mild dehydration can lead to low energy, constipation, dull skin, brittle nails, and

Hydration Tips

Are you wondering how much water to drink? The general recommendation is to drink half your body weight in ounces each day. Use this as a guide, not a hard-and-fast rule. You may need to increase your hydration when in particularly hot environments, after participating in intense exercise, when you're feeling under the weather, when you're traveling, or when you're pregnant or nursing. If you need extra support, 100 percent pure coconut water can be a great way to replace minerals and electrolytes such as potassium, sodium, and magnesium.[11]

suppressed immune function. Many of us stock up on skin-care products, hoping to restore our complexion, while skipping one of the most impactful and simple skin-care hacks of all time: staying hydrated. Drinking water is a key component to nourishing our bodies, from the inside out.

Embracing (and Simplifying) Meal Planning

When I was growing up, my mom planned our family's meals each week, and while she didn't exactly enjoy it, it made her life as a working mom less stressful. She planned a meal for each night of the week so that as she rushed home from work to pick us up in the car pool line or from soccer practice, there was nothing to decide. Planning ahead reduced decision fatigue and prevented frantic rush-hour trips to the grocery store when what she really wanted to do was be with her family.

My mom had a list of (mostly) family-approved recipes and rotated them week by week. Once she decided on the meals for the week, she made her grocery list, writing the items according to where they were in the store so she could get in and out efficiently. I used to think it was incredible that she knew where everything was in the store, but now here I am, meal planning for my family and making my list in order of the grocery store aisles, just like she did.

Maybe you're already an expert-level meal planner, or maybe the phrase alone makes you want to turn and run. I've been on both ends of the spectrum at various points in my life. But I can tell you this: if you want to ensure that you're nourishing your body well, weekly meal planning is one of the easiest and most impactful changes you can make.

This is another area where it's easy to fall into an all-or-nothing mentality. But the reality is, we all do meal planning in some fashion, whether it's a series of hurried daily decisions or a thoughtful, preplanned week.

As we discussed with exercise, it's important to have a plan but to keep it flexible. Depending on your personality or your schedule or the needs of your family, you can plan all your meals, down to the snacks you want to enjoy, or you can simply plan a few meals and foods that you want to have on hand to support your wellness in the midst of a busy week.

Meal Planning and Preparation Tips

Here are a few suggestions to help you feel confident about your meal options and reduce the stress of daily meal preparation:

- **Look at your calendar** for the week and decide which meals you'll eat at home and which ones you'll eat out or at work. This will help you decide how much food to buy and what ingredients you'll need.

- **Go through your list** of meals and choose which ones you'll make for the week, then make a list of the items you need to purchase.

- **If you're short on time** or want to avoid impulse buys, consider using an online grocery ordering or delivery service.

- **As soon as the groceries land in your kitchen,** take a few minutes to wash and prep some veggies and fruits to have on hand for snacks and quick lunches during the week. (This is a great responsibility to delegate to older kids!)

- **If you decide to prepare** a few meals or snacks ahead of time, make it a family affair. Talk to the other people in your household and ask them what they'd like to help prepare for the week ahead. Not only can this activity be good for your relationships, but it also gives family members some owner-ship over meals throughout the week.

- **Cooking for one?** Try planning and prepping a few meals with a friend! You can each prepare a recipe and split it in half to share for the week.

- **Store your prepared foods** in glass containers for ultimate freshness and so you can see them clearly. This makes grabbing a healthy meal or snack an easier choice. As a bonus, you'll reduce exposure to potentially harmful chemicals found in plastic.

- **If meal planning seems overwhelming,** remember that you don't have to map out the entire week in one sitting. Planning just one or two meals can help ensure that you'll feed yourself well, even when life gets busy.

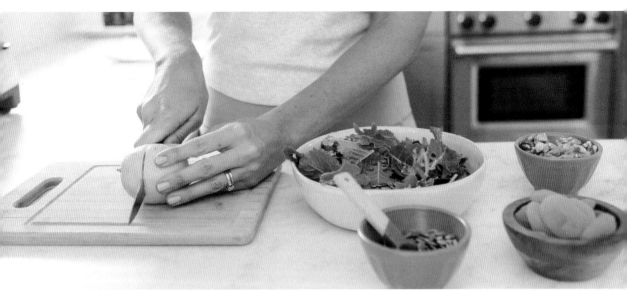

Keep It Simple

I put a high value on the quality of food that I eat and serve to my family. But in order to keep food in its proper place and avoid falling into unhealthy patterns, I don't strive for perfection. While I do my best to fill my family's plates with quality foods throughout the week, it's all about balance. Just today my kids had burgers and fries for lunch followed by a sugary "smoothie" (one that should really be categorized as a milkshake), and I enjoyed a delicious afternoon latte and a bar of dark chocolate. And I have zero stress about it. We'll return to more nourishing foods at our next meal—it's all about balance.

If you notice the all-or-nothing mentality creeping into your food choices, aim for the 80/20 principle: 80 percent of your diet consisting of nourishing, nutrient-rich foods and then allowing some leeway with the other 20 percent. This rhythm helps my family as I cook meals at home with quality ingredients while we also enjoy our favorite restaurants and treats on occasion.

When you allow room in your diet for variety, focusing primarily on foods that nourish you while also celebrating food as a source of pleasure, you'll be better able to practice moderation. When you let go of strict rules and when no foods are off limits (barring allergies or medical needs), the pressure and guilt around food dissipates. This benefits you—and also those around you. The people in your sphere of influence (your children, your partner, your friends, and your extended family) have an opportunity to see what a healthy, balanced relationship with food can look like.

The world of food and nutrition can be overwhelming. As someone who has been in the wellness industry for more than a decade, I've seen trends come and go. New research consistently comes out that challenges what we thought we knew about food and the way it impacts our health. But there are a few things that have stood the test of time and continue to be supported by research and practitioners from a variety of backgrounds.

When it comes to making nutrition choices that are wise and sustainable, it's best to keep it simple: fill your diet with as many whole, anti-inflammatory foods as possible; reduce foods that are fried, highly processed, or high in sugar; and stay hydrated. This will keep your body nourished from the inside out. You are worth caring for and fueling with nourishing foods. One of the best ways to support your well-being and practice self-care is to practice mindfulness about what you put in your body.

For Those Who Don't Have the Luxury of Keeping It Simple

If you have dietary restrictions, whether because of medical needs or food allergies, the task of making decisions around food may seem daunting. In these scenarios, the 80/20 principle may not apply in the same way. For many years, I had a child with severe food allergies and a long list of dietary restrictions to support his health. One thing I learned along the way was how important meal planning was for my family. We didn't have the luxury of going along with whatever was on the menu at events, eating whatever was served at birthday parties, or even participating in the school lunch program. Everywhere we went, we traveled with our own food, and it felt anything but simple, but it was possible if we planned ahead. If you're navigating a similar road, I see you and applaud you for doing what you need to do to care for your needs and the needs of your family.

- **Instead of asking yourself,** *Should I eat this?* consider asking, *Will this provide my body the nourishment it needs?*

- **Make it a goal** to eat at least one food per day that's known to reduce inflammation in the body.

- **When you sit down for a meal,** pause, take a deep breath, and tune in to the present moment to increase mindfulness and improve digestion.

- **When you notice a craving,** make a mental note of where it might be coming from to help you feel more empowered and in control. (Are you bored? Tired? Dehydrated?)

- **Whenever possible,** try to include protein and healthy fat at each meal and snack.

- **Plan at least one nourishing,** nutrient-rich meal for the week ahead. (See the following recipes for a quick, easy idea.)

Bacon and Chickpea Salad with Dairy-Free Ranch Dressing

SERVES: 4

Think salads are boring? Think again! This protein-packed salad is full of flavor from smoky bacon, sweet potatoes, crunchy sprouts, and a dairy-free creamy dressing made with hempseed. This dressing makes about $^2/_3$ cup. It can be doubled and stored in a sealed container in the refrigerator for up to four days. If you don't have time to whip up your own dressing, try Primal Kitchen or Whole30 Ranch.

Salad Ingredients

8 slices (64 g) bacon, sugar-free, if preferred
1 cup (152 g) canned chickpeas, drained
1 large sweet potato, chopped
5 cups (275 g) romaine lettuce, chopped
1 cup (142 g) cucumber, chopped
1 cup (180 g) cherry tomatoes, halved
2 tbsp (18 g) sunflower seeds
1 cup (33 g) alfalfa sprouts

Dressing Ingredients

$^2/_3$ cup (80 g) hempseed
$^1/_2$ cup (118 ml) water
   (plus more, as needed)
1 clove garlic, peeled
1 tsp (2 g) lemon zest
1 tsp (3 g) nutritional yeast
$^1/_2$ tsp (2.5 g) sea salt
$^1/_4$ tsp (.5 g) black pepper
3 tbsp (45 ml) lemon juice
1 tbsp (1 g) dill, chopped
1 tbsp (3 g) chives, chopped
1 tbsp (4 g) parsley, chopped

Preparation

1. Preheat the oven to 400°F (204°C). Line a baking tray with foil.
2. Add bacon to the tray.
3. Bake for 18–22 minutes or until bacon is crispy. Remove bacon and set aside. Once cool, crumble into bite-size pieces.
4. Add chickpeas and potatoes to the baking tray, mixing to combine. Season with salt and pepper.
5. Bake for 20–30 minutes or until potatoes are tender and chickpeas are crispy. Let cool.

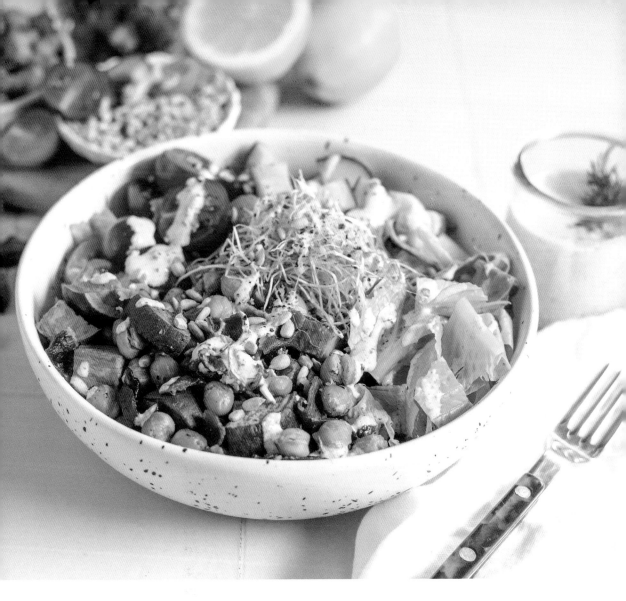

6. Meanwhile, make the dressing. Combine the hempseed, water, garlic, lemon zest, nutritional yeast, salt, pepper, and lemon juice in a high-speed blender. Add water as needed, one tablespoon at a time, to help the mixture blend together.

7. Once the mixture is smooth, stir in the dill, chives, and parsley.

8. To assemble, divide the romaine into four bowls. Top with bacon, chick-peas, sweet potato, cucumber, and tomato. Garnish with sunflower seeds and alfalfa sprouts.

9. Drizzle ranch dressing over the top, and enjoy!

One-Pan Chicken Fajitas with Mango Salsa

SERVES: 4

Make a dinner the whole family will love—and you'll love the easy cleanup! This one-pan meal is the perfect weeknight dinner, as it's on the table in less than forty-five minutes! If you're looking for a different protein option, you can substitute chicken for chickpeas or tofu for a meatless meal. I love using Siete grain-free tortillas (the almond flour provides additional protein and healthy fats), but feel free to use the tortillas you like best. If you don't have fresh mango, you can substitute one cup frozen mango.

Fajita Ingredients

1 lb (454 g) chicken breast, cut into strips
2 medium bell peppers, cut into strips
2 medium zucchini/courgettes, sliced into sticks
1 medium red onion, sliced
2 tsp (5 g) chili powder
1 ½ tsp (3 g) ground cumin
1 tsp (2 g) ground coriander
1 tsp (2 g) smoked paprika
1 tsp (3 g) garlic powder
½ tsp (.5 g) oregano
sea salt and pepper, to taste
2 tbsp (30 ml) olive oil
¼ cup (4 g) cilantro or coriander, chopped
juice of 1 lime

Salsa Ingredients

1 large mango, peeled and chopped
2 tbsp (6 g) red onion, chopped
2 tbsp (2 g) fresh cilantro or coriander, chopped
2 tsp (30 g) finely chopped jalapeño, seeds removed
juice of one lime
sea salt, to taste

Serving Ingredients

8 grain-free tortillas
fresh mango salsa (recipe above)
1 avocado, sliced
2 limes, cut into wedges
plain coconut yogurt or Greek yogurt, optional

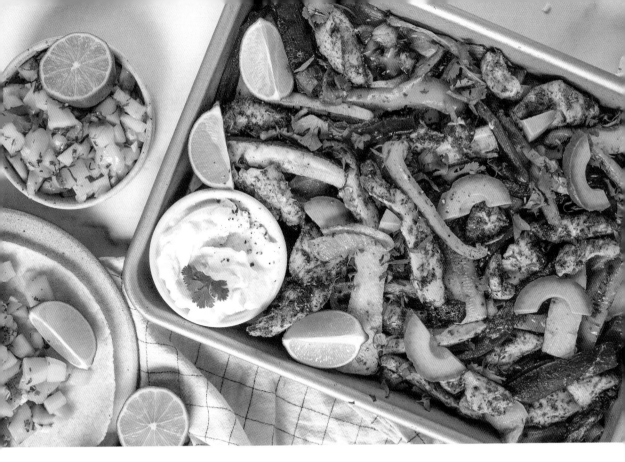

Preparation

1. Preheat the oven to 425°F (218°C). Line a baking tray with foil.
2. Add the chicken, peppers, zucchini, and onion to a large bowl.
3. Combine chili powder, cumin, coriander, smoked paprika, garlic powder, oregano, salt, and pepper with the olive oil, and pour over chicken and veggies. Mix until evenly distributed.
4. Add the chicken mixture to a baking tray in a single layer.
5. Bake for 22–27 minutes, or until the chicken is completely baked through and the vegetables are tender.
6. Top with cilantro and lime juice.
7. While the chicken is cooking, make the mango salsa. Combine mango, red onion, cilantro, jalapeño, and lime juice in a bowl. Season with sea salt.
8. To assemble, serve the chicken mixture in grain-free tortillas (or in a salad) with mango salsa, avocado, lime wedges, and yogurt.

Blueberry Almond Smoothie

SERVES: 1

With a healthy dose of protein and nourishing fats from almond butter and chia seeds, this smoothie will help you power through your morning routine. Chia seeds are a great way to add heart-healthy omega-3 fatty acids and fiber to your diet. Hempseed provides omega-3 fatty acids and protein, as well as relaxing magnesium.

Ingredients

³/₄ **cup (177 ml)** coconut water

³/₄ **cup (142 g)** frozen blueberries

¹/₂ **medium** banana, frozen

1 tbsp (16 g) almond butter

2 tsp (6 g) chia seeds

3 tbsp (30 g) hempseed, optional

Preparation

1. Combine all ingredients in a high-speed blender until smooth.
2. Enjoy immediately.

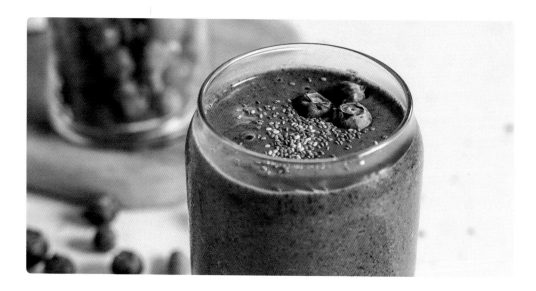

Chapter 4

listen

If you are not aware
of what your body
needs, you can't
take care of it.

Bessel van der Kolk

What does your body need right now?

No, really. Pause, take a big inhale, then exhale slowly. Scan your body to see what it's telling you in this moment.

If this is the first time you've stopped to ask your body what it needs, this may feel foreign at first. Many of us learned from a young age to ignore or override our bodies' cues. We were taught to listen to our elders because they knew better than we did. We were told to finish the food on our plates even if we were no longer hungry. We were taught to wait until bathroom breaks to use the restroom.

As adults, we follow diets that teach

us to ignore our hunger, urging us to muster up enough willpower to override our cravings or the sensation of hunger. Meanwhile, we listen to fitness instructors who shout at us to push through the pain while ignoring what our bodies are telling us. Messages such as "No pain, no gain" and "Mind over matter" pervade the fitness world.

Without realizing it, we've grown accustomed to silencing the body's cues and ignoring its needs in an effort to "be good," and as a result, we've lost the ability to trust ourselves. Our bodies and our minds have become strangers at best and enemies at worst.

As a culture, we've shifted away from listening to our unique needs while habitually looking elsewhere for guidance. This tendency to delegate choices about our health is understandable. Our plates are full, our schedules are tight, and almost everything we need is just a Google search away (or at least it seems that way). Add to that the years we've spent following prescriptive diets and workout plans that told us exactly what we needed to do to be "healthy," and it's no wonder we're out of touch with what our bodies really need at any given moment.

As we discussed in chapter 2, the secret to health is learning to work with our bodies, rather than against them. This means that instead of pushing through the pain, we notice when something doesn't feel right and then adjust accordingly.

One of the benefits of Pilates is that it can be modified to support any type of body and any set of circumstances. So instead of trying to fit your body into an existing mold or system, you can adapt the exercises to support your individual needs. I encourage my clients to understand that modifying is not seen as cheating. Instead, it's a necessary way to get the most out of each exercise.

The truth is, the body regularly sends us messages about what it wants and needs. Unfortunately, it's easy to lose (or never develop) the ability to hear what it's saying.

Honoring the Season You're In

We are often so inundated with information about what's happening around us—from news outlets, advertisements, podcasts, and social media—that it's hard to hear what our bodies want us to hear. So with all the noise around us, how can we begin to tune in to our bodies' needs?

One practical way to quiet the outside voices is to take an honest look at your

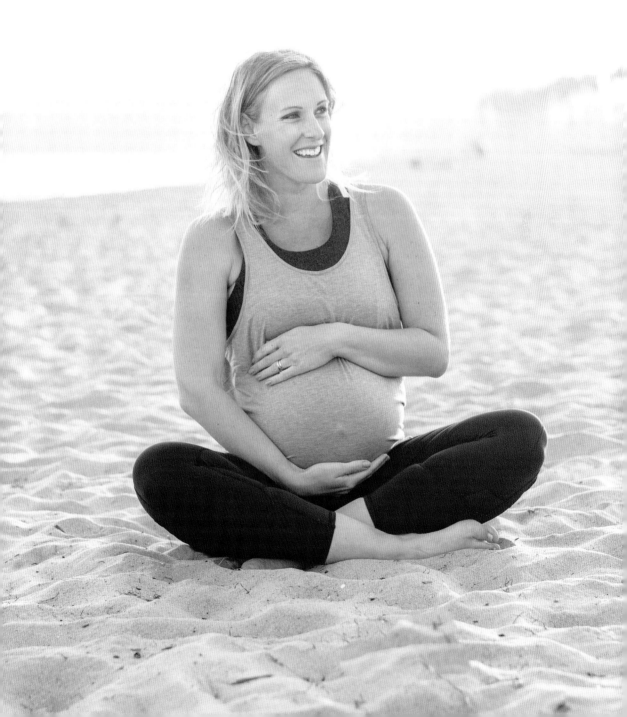

life today—not where you were five years ago or where you want to be in the future, but where you are right now, in your current season of life. What do your days look like? How do you spend your time? What are your current responsibilities? How do those commitments impact your sense of well-being?

The circumstances of my life have changed dramatically over the past decade or so. Fifteen years ago, I was living in California, dating Matt, and living in an old house with four of my best friends. I was working my first official full-time job and experiencing crippling anxiety. Every day I was consumed by irrational fears. I was paranoid, imagining threats at nearly every turn.

A few years later, I was married to Matt and living in Colorado. We were expecting our first baby, and we weren't sure how we'd pay the bills each month. I never could have guessed that five years later we'd be back in California, juggling four kids under the age of six, and I'd be the CEO of a fast-growing company. Within each of those broader seasons were smaller ones too—seasons of pregnancy, postpartum, loss, recovery, health challenges, healing, grief, celebration, and even wildfires and mudslides.

While your details will look different from mine, you've been through seasons of your own, and you're in a unique season right now. If we don't take time to pause

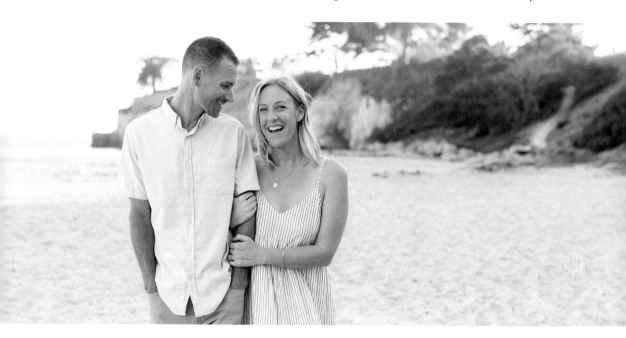

and acknowledge our current circumstances, we'll make the mistake of assuming that what our minds and bodies needed in the past is the same thing we need right now. We end up making decisions based on a season we're no longer in—decisions that are no longer ideal for our current reality.

In order to connect to our bodies, we must acknowledge that they can change.

Even when we're facing something we've been through before, there are unique circumstances that set each experience apart. For me, this became especially apparent after each of my pregnancies. A few months after having my first baby, I started training for a half-marathon. I had the energy, I felt great physically, my schedule allowed for it, and I liked how strong it made me feel. I worked hard, pushed myself, and went for countless runs with my baby napping in the stroller. On race day, I nursed my daughter at the starting line, passed her off to a friend, ran the race, and then nursed her at the finish line with sweat dripping down my face.

Fast-forward to a later postpartum season, when I had a five-year-old, a three-year-old, and newborn twins. I was nursing two babies around the clock, my energy was down, my body was depleted of nutrients, and my physical recovery was much slower (hello, two placentas, two babies, and two deliveries nine minutes apart). Training for a half-marathon in that season of my life would have been detrimental to my well-being. Any spare time I had was best used for resting, feeding myself, showering, and calming my nervous system. I was healing diastasis recti (separation along the abdominal muscles as a result of pregnancy) and reconnecting with my pelvic floor, and the majority of my energy was going toward keeping my children alive and well. That time around, returning to exercise was an extremely slow and gentle process.

What "healthy" looked like for you ten years ago will look different from the way it looks in your current season—and that's okay. It's tempting to compare yourself to where you were in a previous season, whether that's a number on the scale, a pant size, or a certain level of fitness. We often beat ourselves up, saying, *I used to be able to do that; why can't I do it now?* But transitions are a natural part of life. From puberty to hormonal fluctuations to pregnancy to menopause, our seasons change. In order to connect to our bodies, we must acknowledge that they can change.

A few months after the twins were born, I faced an unexpected challenge that forced me to look at healthy choices in a whole new way. I once assumed cardio workouts that spiked my heart rate and challenged my stamina were always good for me. I used to enjoy long runs, and I would add high-intensity interval training to my workout routine for extra cardio benefit.

But after meeting with doctors and getting a better understanding of my health during that season, I saw that high-intensity workouts were hurting more than they were helping. As a result of chronic stress and what turned out to be high levels of mycotoxins in my system from mold exposure, my hormones were completely out of balance. My cortisol, estrogen, and progesterone levels were so far below normal that they were nearly undetectable.

High-intensity interval training workouts, which include ten- to sixty-second bursts of intense activity followed by a rest period of about the same length, and other forms of high-intensity exercise spike cortisol levels and act as an acute form of stress on the body.[1] When the body is functioning optimally, this can be a good thing! By putting your body through a little stress, you can experience positive physiological benefits, such as increased metabolism, improved insulin sensitivity, and reduction in body fat.[2] When my hormones were in balance, high-intensity

interval training (HIIT) workouts were a healthy choice for me. But when my corti-sol levels were out of balance, my high-intensity workouts were actually having a harmful impact on my hormones.[3]

In hindsight, I can see that when I started doing these intense workouts, I began to get sick more often and felt more run down than energized. It was a frustrat-ing cycle—I'd be motivated to start working out harder and pushing myself in new ways, and within a week, I'd be out with a cold, or my energy would be so low that I couldn't stay consistent.

Eventually, I tuned in to my body and recognized that something wasn't right. When I saw the pattern of feeling worse, not better, after certain workouts, I was able to accept that my whole understanding of what was healthy for me in that sea-son needed to change. While pushing myself hard and prioritizing early-morning workouts would have been a healthy choice five years earlier, I needed to dial it back. In that season, prioritizing sleep was the best thing I could do to support my health and healing. (I discovered that for me, Pilates and walking were the perfect combination—and they still are!)

Maybe you're in a season when you can go for long runs and push yourself toward challenging goals. Or maybe you're working two jobs to make ends meet,

Accepting the season you're in is incredibly freeing and helpful in your journey to be well.

so the best thing you can do is to focus on what's reasonable within your existing routine. Maybe you're pregnant or nursing or going through menopause. Or maybe you're in a season of stress and you need to prioritize sleep, reduce pressure on yourself, and restore peace to your body and mind.

It may sound like a downer that the needs of your body shift, but it's actually good news! Accepting the season you're in is incredibly freeing and helpful in your journey to be well. The truth is, circumstances change. We change. Our bodies change. This is a normal part of life, not something to resist. Instead of looking back and comparing your current self to a past version of yourself, tune in to where you are today and use that as a guide for moving forward.

Learning to Trust Yourself Again

When my husband and I were debating whether we should attempt to grow our family beyond two kids, I talked to friends, prayed, and had deep conversations with Matt. And when those sources weren't giving me a clear answer, I turned to the Internet. Yes, I'm 100 percent embarrassed to admit that I googled (possibly on multiple occasions), "Should I have a third kid?"

I figured someone out there had probably written about their experience of going from two to three kids, and perhaps in a random stranger's blog post I would find the answer I was looking for. I realize this is ridiculous, but it was such a habit for me to search for answers on Google that I did exactly that.

This habit of looking "out there" for answers about what's best for us is something that creeps in over time. We turn to articles to tell us what to wear and what not to wear based on our body types. We watch morning shows that tell us to eat this and not that. We follow influencers and experts on social media, all in the hope of finding the next quick tip that will help us get where we want to be.

It's incredible to be able to connect with smart, inspiring people we never had access to before. I enjoy learning tips, tricks, and strategies that make my life better, and I love being able to share my area of expertise to help others as well. But if we're not careful, we begin to trust the many voices we hear throughout the day above our own. We become so accustomed to seeking answers from other people and finding out what worked for them that we forget to tune in to what we need—in our individual lives, with our unique bodies, minds, and circumstances.

Whether you realize it or not, your body is talking to you. If you're not sure what it's telling you, it may be time to quiet the outside noise and tune in to find out.

So where do you begin? The first step is to learn to trust yourself. Think of intuition as a muscle. The more you listen to your body, the more skilled you get and the easier it becomes.

Practical Ways to Tune In

There are two steps to this skill of listening to your body: first, acknowledge what your body needs, and second, respond to and honor those needs. You may be aware that something needs attention (step one), but things break down when it comes to taking action (step two).

Perhaps deep down you know you need some time to unplug, be alone, or sleep, but you've been ignoring that need because it seems inconvenient, selfish, indulgent, or even impossible. Or perhaps that nagging pain in your back has become so familiar that, while you're aware of it, it's no longer on your radar to do anything about it. Our bodies send us cues, large and small, throughout the day. Some of these we naturally honor, some we unknowingly overlook, and some we intentionally ignore.

Here are some practical ways to build the habit of listening to your body. As you go through your day, tune in to the following cues and then respond appropriately whenever you can.

Thirst: Notice when you feel the physical sensation of thirst (step one). Instead of continuing what you're doing or grabbing another cup of coffee, pause, get some water, and respond to your body's need for hydration (step two). Bonus points if you take a moment to be grateful for access to clean water—what a gift!

Using the restroom: This might seem silly at first, but it's a small, practical way you can tune in to what your body needs. When you're in a busy season, you may notice that you need to use the restroom but ignore the sensation so you can finish one more task, send one more text, write one more paragraph (currently guilty!), or accommodate someone else's needs. When your body is giving you a cue to use the restroom, practice honoring it as promptly as possible. (Some work or school environments can make this challenging, but just do the best you can.) If you're staying hydrated (good for you!), you'll have plenty of opportunities to practice this throughout the day. On a related note, regular bowel movements are important for good health. Pay attention to your daily habits, and if something seems amiss, take a deeper look at what might be causing the issue or follow up with a health professional.

Hunger and satiety: If you have a complicated relationship with food or if you've spent years dieting, restricting, or bingeing, it can be challenging to know when you're full. Don't be discouraged—this isn't an overnight process, and it's all about progress, not perfection. You can begin to build this skill simply by noticing feelings of hunger throughout the day. Before sitting down to a meal, gauge your level of hunger. When you eat, slow down and pay attention to when you feel satisfied—not overly stuffed, but satiated, meaning the physical feeling of hunger is no longer present. This is hard to do when there are distractions such as TV, work, or your phone, so whenever possible, remove distractions and be present to the meal you're enjoying. Give yourself plenty of grace as you tune in to these biological cues that may not come naturally at first to notice.

Tension: Notice when your body feels stiff or tense. Instead of carrying on with the task at hand or habitually popping a pain reliever, pause and respond. That might look like getting up from your desk and walking around to increase blood flow, doing a few stretches to loosen up tight muscles, booking a massage or a chiropractor appointment, or making a plan to incorporate Pilates into your workout routine that week. (See the end of this chapter for a quick, effective Pilates routine you can do at home.)

Exhaustion: When you notice that you're exhausted, what do you do? Do you grab an extra cup of coffee, push through the day, and accept that this is just the way it is? The next time you feel wiped out, notice how your body feels and consider how you can respond given the circumstances. If you're short on time, this may be as simple as lying down to do five minutes of breathing before your next meeting (see chapter 8 for a quick breathing exercise) or stepping outside for a bit of fresh air and sunshine. Or it might be a cue to make some bigger changes, such as reworking your schedule, hiring help, or pruning your commitments. Only you know what's best, and only you can give your body what it needs. Your health depends on it.

Pilates as a Method of Listening

During a Pilates workout, you learn to pay attention to the way your body feels as you move through different exercises. You begin to notice where you are in space, the position of your body, and how to adjust, adapt, engage, and release. You discover how to breathe with intention and release tension, using your body weight to build strength and endurance.

Instead of being distracted by blaring music or being entertained by instructors so you forget the pain, doing Pilates requires presence, focus, and concentration.

I often begin the classes I teach by encouraging students to scan their bodies from head to toe, simply taking note of how they feel that day. When I do this myself, I'm always surprised by what I find. I may notice a spot of tension I've been holding in my neck or a bit of tightness in my lower back. I may notice that my energy is lower than usual or I'm a bit under the weather. Practicing Pilates is a practical way to restore the connection between your mind and your body, which makes it easier to notice when your body is speaking to you.

A Note about Trauma

Traumatic experiences can have a significant impact on our ability to inhabit our bodies. If you've experienced trauma, know that you're not alone and there are resources available to help you. Pilates can help, but you may also want to find a professional to help you with cognitive behavioral therapy, EMDR (eye movement desensitization and reprocessing), neurofeedback, or EFT (emotional freedom technique). *The Body Keeps the Score* by Besser van der Kolk may be a helpful resource as well.

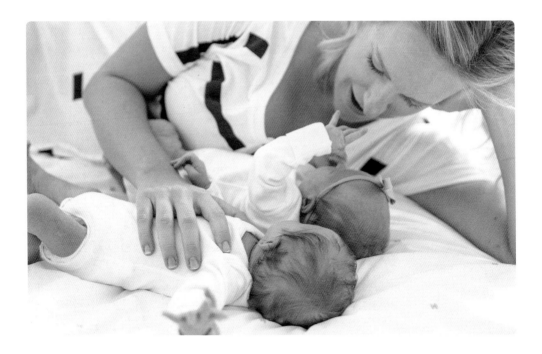

The Importance of Listening and Responding

In *The Body Keeps the Score*, a groundbreaking book that discusses the healing of trauma in the brain, mind, and body, Besser van der Kolk says, "One of the clearest lessons from contemporary neuroscience is that our sense of ourselves is anchored in a vital connection with our bodies. We do not truly know ourselves unless we can feel and interpret our physical sensations; we need to register and act on these sensations to navigate safely through life." When we acknowledge what we're feeling and act on it, we're able to connect with our bodies and make peace with our bodies. This is a necessary part of being fully alive. Van der Kolk goes on to say, "While numbing (or compensatory sensation seeking) may make life tolerable, the price you pay is that you lose awareness of what is going on inside your body and, with that, the sense of being fully, sensually alive."[4]

Shortly after the birth of my twins, I had an inkling that something was off in my body, but I continued to downplay my symptoms. When I felt exhausted and achy, I'd chalk it up to a bad night of sleep or something I ate. I reasoned that my joints were sore due to my office chair, or I figured my muscles were stiff because I was too cold throughout the day.

It wasn't until a morning in January, when I was getting ready for the day, brushing my thinning hair and limping to my closet in pain, that I finally paused and allowed myself to acknowledge the inner voice that was telling me something was truly wrong. I recognized that the way I was feeling was not normal, and I could no longer ignore what my body was telling me.

Later that evening, when I told my husband I was (once again) too tired to talk after the kids were in bed and I collapsed onto the couch, he expressed his concern that he never saw me *not* tired anymore. In that moment, I knew it was well past time to take the messages from my body seriously.

It took months of doctor visits, multiple phone calls, and research for me to get a handle on what was causing my symptoms. Through various tests, my doctor discovered that I had high levels of mycotoxins in my body as a result of exposure to mold in a previous home, as well as extremely low hormone levels, likely due to chronic stress. When she saw my results, she looked me in the eye and said, "I'm amazed you're even able to get out of bed."

It's been a few years since that doctor appointment, and while I may never know for certain what caused all my symptoms, I'm grateful that I listened to my body's needs and responded with action to begin a path toward healing.

When I shared this story on my podcast, I was blown away by the response. I figured I'd hear from listeners with questions about my symptoms or what I was doing to recover, but to my surprise, most of the messages said, "Thank you—this is the nudge I needed to listen to my body too."

I understand the desire to sweep health concerns under the rug. Acknowledging that something doesn't feel right can be inconvenient at best and terrifying at worst. When I was experiencing symptoms of my own, I didn't feel like I had the time, energy, or bandwidth to advocate for myself and take the next steps. I also didn't know where to start.

So many factors can hold us back from seeking help, including budget concerns, access to quality care, having the time to go to appointments, or even our own ego. We also have a tendency to delegate our health decisions to someone else—a doctor, a parent, or a spouse. But if we don't advocate for our own well-being, we may miss early detection opportunities, suffer unnecessarily, or further damage our mental and physical health.

I'm incredibly grateful that I was able to get the help I needed and receive care (a privilege I don't take lightly). The ability to listen to our bodies and advocate for our health is something that will serve us on a daily basis, as well as for a lifetime. Staying aware of our physical, mental, and emotional needs isn't always easy or convenient, but it's always worth it.

〰 Put It into Practice

- **Input calendar reminders** to pop up a few times throughout the day to remind you to take a few deep breaths and mentally scan your body to see how it feels. When you notice something that needs attention, respond accordingly.

- **The next time you notice you need to use the restroom,** stop what you're doing and go! (And if you notice you haven't gone in a while, pay attention to that, too.)

- **At the beginning of your next meal,** pause to notice your level of physical hunger. Pause again in the middle of your meal, and then notice how you feel when you're done. Are you satisfied? Still hungry? Stuffed? This isn't about guilt or shame, just about paying attention.

- **Add at least one Pilates workout** to your weekly routine to help you build the skill of reconnecting to your body in new and positive ways.

- **Write in your journal.** Is there anything your body has been telling you that you've been ignoring? Write about it. Even if you don't know how to respond yet, taking time to reconnect with what your body is telling you will move you forward on your journey.

Pilates Workout

 This ten-minute Pilates workout is designed to help you develop the skill of listening to your body. Through breathing, stretching, and verbal cues, I guide you through a series of exercises to leave you feeling more connected to your body and to what you truly need. Scan the QR code to access the video of this gentle and effective workout.

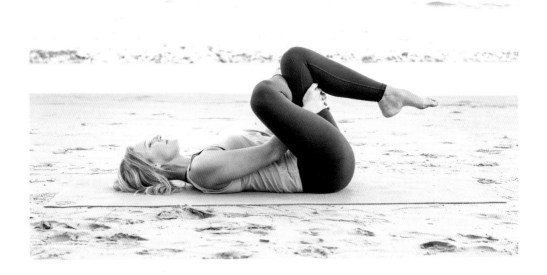

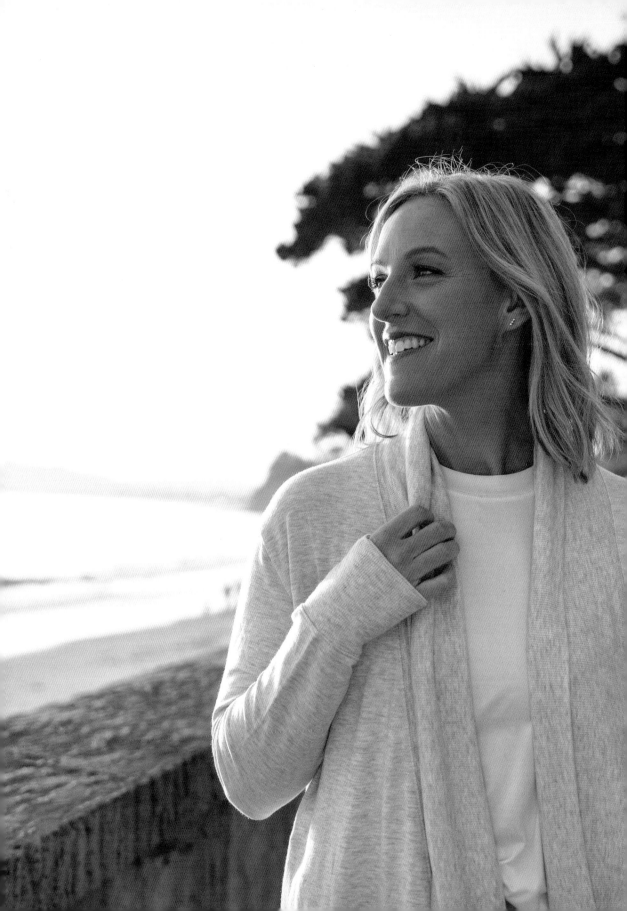

unplug

Almost everything
will work again
if you unplug it
for a few minutes,
including you.

Anne Lamott

We live in a hyperconnected world. I don't know about you, but the majority of my day involves some form of technology. Whether I'm texting with a friend, sending an email for work, calling my mom, listening to a podcast, ordering groceries, or shopping for new furniture, it all happens digitally.

I'm incredibly grateful for the gift of technology. Not only does it keep me informed and allow me to order dinner for my family with the click of a button, but it has also made it possible for me to build a business that supports women all over the world and provide jobs for my incredible team members, who benefit from the opportunity to work from home. So don't worry—I'm not here to tell you to toss your devices and live off the grid. But I would like to reveal some eye-opening ways our relationship with technology may impact our health and well-being.

In a recent study on smartphone use, nearly half of the respondents stated that they spend, on average, five to six hours per day on their phones (not including work-related tasks).[1] With computer and television use factored in, it's clear that the majority of our days are spent connected to a device.

Nearly every part of our lives has some digital component. Even when I'm cooking, I often look at a recipe on an app on my phone while pulling up a playlist on our smart home device. Technology has revolutionized the way we live. But do we ever stop to ask ourselves, *At what cost?*

In this chapter we'll navigate what it looks like to have a healthy relationship with technology and how to replace what has been lost as a result of our screen-centric lifestyle.

Anxiety and Information Overload

Have you ever felt overwhelmed when spending time online, perhaps after scrolling through social media or catching up on the news? Information overload is real. We click on an eye-catching headline, a politically charged news piece, or a heartbreaking Instagram post, and all at once we're inundated with information.

We want to be informed; we want to know what's going on; we want to see what other people are saying. But as it turns out, we weren't designed to live this way. We weren't made to carry the weight of the world, quite literally, in the palm of our hand. Whether we realize it or not, this constant influx of information takes a toll on our mental and physical health.

Cell phone use alone has been connected to the following side effects:

- a decrease in attention span[2]

- an increase in anxiety and depression

- sleep disturbances

- heightened stress response and increased stress hormones

- reduced brain function[3]

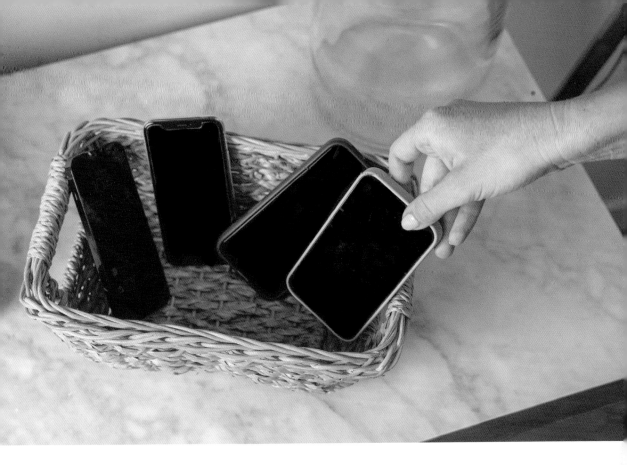

- increased oxidative stress (which can lead to illness and disease)[4]

- neck and back pain

- vision impairment

- increased risk of traffic incidents[5]

What's more, cell phone addiction is real.[6] I will be the first person to tell you I have a problem, and I've been working on it. If I'm not intentional about boundaries, I will habitually check my phone throughout the day, even if I don't have a reason to. I'll look up a recipe, and all of a sudden I'm scrolling through Instagram without even knowing how I got there! Even when I'm tired and want to go to bed, I'll keep looking at my phone. This isn't the way I want to live. I told my oldest daughter (only half joking) that she's not allowed to have a phone until her dad and I can figure out how to model a healthier relationship with our phones. She is now heavily invested in my efforts, and the extra accountability is actually quite helpful.

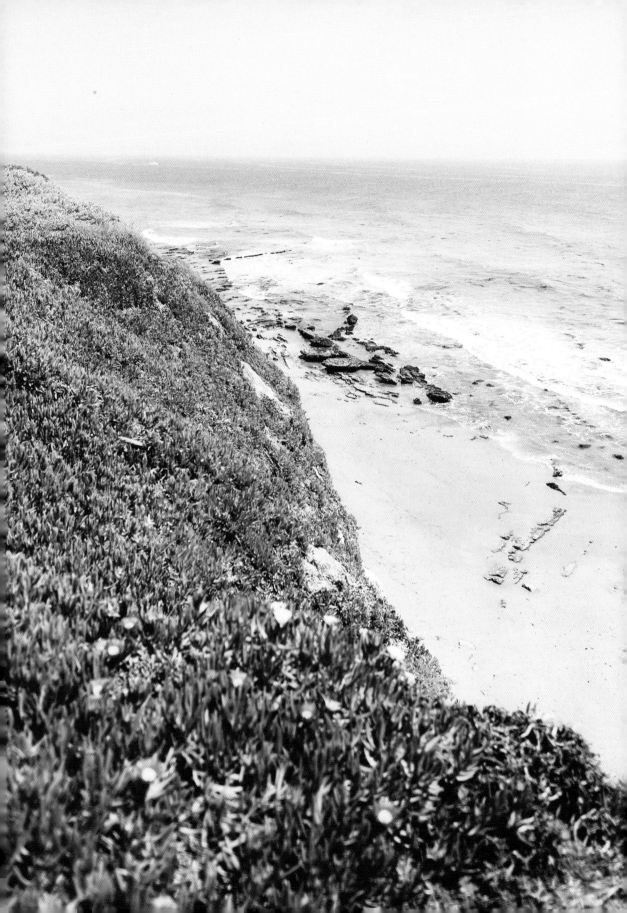

Cell phones and, more specifically, the apps we use on them are designed to hook us. They're strategically engineered to trigger our brains to release dopamine (the pleasure hormone) to keep us coming back for more, making it extremely hard to not check our phones and open our apps repeatedly throughout the day. When you take notifications into account, it becomes nearly impossible not to just take a peek to see what has popped up since you last checked.

As a mother (and as someone who greatly cares about the upcoming generation of humans), I find the impact of cell phones on the mental health of children and teenagers deeply concerning. In his book *Digital Minimalism*, Cal Newport discusses the impact of constant digital connection on teenagers. "Teenagers have lost the ability to process and make sense of their emotions, or to reflect on who they are and what really matters, or to build strong relationships, or even to just allow their brains time to power down their critical social circuits, which are not meant to be used constantly, and to redirect that energy to other important cognitive housekeeping tasks. We shouldn't be surprised that these absences lead to malfunctions."[7]

Study after study shows that smartphones, social media, and screen time in general are related to increased rates of depression, anxiety, and suicidal thoughts in young people. When we consider the physical and mental impact of looking at screens all day and being overloaded with information every time we pick up our phones, it's clear that something needs to change.

Yes, this information is sobering, but we don't need to feel hopeless or paralyzed. As you know by now, small changes can make a huge impact. We don't have to go to extremes in order to improve our well-being.

I'm starting at home, with myself. I'm learning to model a healthy relationship with technology, and I hope you'll join me.

Creating Pockets of Silence

When I first discovered that chronic stress was a factor in my hormonal imbalance, I was confused. Sure, my life was incredibly full at the time, but I didn't *feel* stressed on a daily basis. I was busy, but I was managing. Or so I thought.

My medical crisis forced me to take a hard look at my habits, and one of my key realizations was that I was living in a constant state of stimulation. The input was nonstop. Whether it was an incoming email, a text from a friend, a crying baby, a yelling toddler, a ringing doorbell, or a news headline on the current state of the world, I was constantly surrounded by stimulation.

The increase in input was gradual and happened over a span of years, so my brain adapted as well as it could . . . until it reached a breaking point. Without realizing it, I was living in a constant state of fight or flight. My nervous system was on overdrive, and my mental and physical health were declining as a result. It was sneaky and subtle—until it wasn't.

While we can't control everything that comes our way each day, we can be intentional about reducing our input to allow our minds to process information and our nervous systems to regulate.

At the height of my overwhelm, I started thinking about ways I could reduce my stimulation throughout the day. I set out to create more pockets of silence, even if just for a few minutes at a time. Instead of scrolling my phone while nursing one of the twins, I left it in the other room, closed my eyes, took deep breaths, and allowed myself to think without any additional input. While driving in the car, instead of instinctively putting on music or a podcast, I'd consider whether silence would better fit my needs that day. I started going for fifteen-minute walks in the morning while leaving my phone and headphones at home. I listened to the birds, allowed my mind to wander, and recharged my mental and physical batteries by turning down the volume of life for a few minutes.

The Body's Natural Rhythms

A growing body of research points to the importance of our bodies' natural circadian rhythms and the ways our modern lifestyle disrupts this important biological process.[8] Put simply, the circadian rhythm is the body's twenty-four-hour sleep and wake cycle. While we view waking up and going to bed as basic parts of our day, there's a sophisticated process taking place in the body that impacts everything from our sleep to our energy level, behavior, hormones, and immune system.

The circadian rhythm is essentially the body's internal clock (controlled by the brain) that tells our bodies when to decrease melatonin production as the sun rises (time to wake up!), when to produce proteins in the digestive system according to typical mealtimes (time to digest), and when to release hormones to optimize other important bodily functions throughout the day (time to wind down).

So, what does this have to do with unplugging? Circadian rhythms are controlled

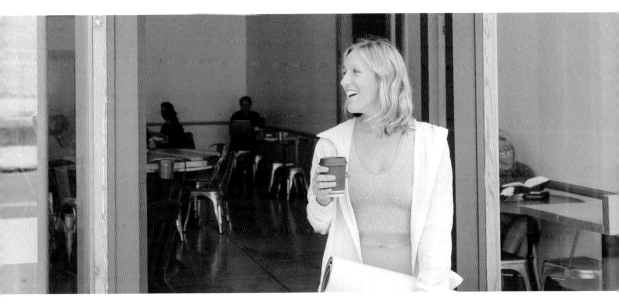

by a part of the brain that's highly sensitive to light (to be specific, the supra-chiasmatic nucleus). Once the brain registers the amount of light in the environment, it uses this information to operate nearly every system and process in the body. (Aren't our bodies incredible?)

Our circadian rhythms rely on being exposed to sunlight in the morning as our bodies stop the production of melatonin and kick-start daily functions. In the evening, as the sun sets and the retina detects less light, our bodies know that it's time to wind down and prepare for sleep by increasing melatonin production.

Let's take a quick look at a fairly typical daily routine:

6:00 a.m.: Wake up, check phone, and get ready for the day

8:00 a.m.: Brief walk to car/transit to commute to work/school (if working from home, go straight to desk)

12:00 p.m.: After hours of sitting at a desk, quick lunch break while sitting (or eating lunch while working)

5:00 p.m.: Drive home to make/eat dinner

8:00 p.m.: Unwind while watching a show, scrolling social media, and/or finishing working on the computer

As you think about this schedule as it relates to the body's natural circadian rhythms, what do you notice? First, there's very little exposure to sunlight in the morning. It's common for many of us to stay indoors during our morning routine—and to spend the majority of the day indoors as well. We miss the crucial step of going outside to get sunlight on our eyes. In doing so, our brains may not fully get the signal that it's time to wake up and jump-start the biological processes that support our mood, energy, digestion, and immune function throughout the day.

Additionally, the evening hours are spent looking at screens, which can send conflicting signals to the brain. Remember, exposure to light affects the biological processes in the body. That means daylight, but it also includes light from screens. In the evening hours, our bodies need to wind down. When we expose the retina to a steady stream of light from screens (aka blue light), this can interfere with the body's ability to release melatonin and prepare for a night of sleep, rest, and recovery.[9]

When my first two children were four and two, I found myself in a stressful season. Weeks after finding out I was pregnant with our third baby, I miscarried. I was devastated and scared. I felt weak and tired, and I did my best to nurture myself back to health. But I was surprised by the lack of support and information for women recovering from miscarriage.

A few months after the loss, I was still feeling off, and I wanted assurance that my hormones were returning to appropriate levels and that my diet was providing adequate nutrition. Not knowing where to turn, I reached out to a nutritionist friend who supported women through the childbearing years.

She had me take a test that analyzed saliva samples from when I woke up, in the midmorning, in the midafternoon, in the evening, and at bedtime. The test was intended to monitor my levels of cortisol throughout the day.

When the nutritionist got my results, she called me to set up a meeting. As soon as we sat down for lunch at an outdoor courtyard, she said, "I have a question for you. Are you working at night after you put the kids in bed?"

That struck me as an odd thing to ask. At the time, I wasn't sure what that had to do with my hormone levels. But I told her that, yes, most nights I put the kids to bed and then opened my laptop to finish work I hadn't been able to complete during the day.

She pulled out my test results and showed me a graph that depicted my cortisol levels. Upon waking up, when my cortisol should have been rising, it was low. In the evening, when my cortisol should have been decreasing in preparation for sleep, it was spiking. These issues were directly related to my morning and evening routines: a lack of daylight in the waking hours (and a body that wasn't recharging properly) and too much screen time and stimulation in the evenings.

Our constant connection to screens affects our health in significant ways that we're often not even aware of. Screen time can disrupt our sleep, impact our hormones, impair digestion, and zap our energy. The good news is that we can take simple steps to break this cycle. One of the most effective ways to break an old habit is to create new rhythms and routines that support the results we desire.

After meeting with my nutritionist, I took a good look at my work schedule and got honest about what was realistic for me to do in a given day. I know I needed to carve out some intentional space for quiet in my daily routine. This will look different for everyone, but here's what it looked like for me. I needed to be intentional about time management, say no to certain things, and have discussions with my team about my capacity and about schedule changes I needed to make so I could slow down and reduce stress. I also implemented an evening routine so I wouldn't default to screen time at night. After putting the kids to bed, I would do one quick check of my messages and then shut down my devices for the night. I began taking nightly baths with Epsom salts to promote relaxation. Instead of looking at screens, I read books so I could truly wind down.

> The goal isn't to be perfect
> but simply to become more intentional
> about how I use technology.

I still love my phone, and I have children who fill our house with an excessive amount of noise and stimulation. But intentionally creating pockets of white space throughout my day and paying attention to my circadian rhythms has helped me to feel better physically, think more clearly, lead more confidently, and parent more calmly. The goal isn't to be perfect but simply to become more intentional about how I use technology.

Think of it like a door that can be opened and closed. When we open social media apps, turn on the news, or press play on a podcast, we're opening the door for information and stimulation to flow into our minds and lives. We can—and must—be intentional about closing that door on occasion to allow our minds to simply *be*—to process, think, tune in to the present moment, listen to our bodies, and focus our attention on what matters most.

Optimizing Your Morning and Evening Routines

Whether you're someone who enjoys structure or someone who doesn't like to feel boxed in, keep in mind that we all have routines—it's just that some people are more intentional about them than others.

You may not realize it, but there are many things you do consistently when you wake up each morning or before you go to bed each evening. Your routines can be as simple or as elaborate as you want them to be; the key is to create a pattern that supports your body's natural circadian rhythms, fosters a healthy relationship with technology, and gives you an overall sense of well-being.

When you're creating (or modifying) a morning and evening routine, here are a few things to think through:

- What are your current morning and evening routines (in other words, the habits you repeat on a regular basis)?

- How are your routines serving you? What's going well? What isn't working for you?

Working the Night Shift?

If you work in the evening or overnight, or if you have a rotating schedule, it can be difficult to feel fully rested and get adequate sleep. If it's possible, it might be worth considering making a change so your schedule can better align with your body's natural rhythms. If that's not an option right now, make use of naps and black-out shades, and try to maintain a consistent sleep schedule whenever you can.[10]

- How much time do you have in the morning before you need to be "on" for the day?

- How much time do you have in the evening before bedtime?

- Do you prefer long, meaningful routines? Or are short, intentional routines better for the season you're in right now?

A few tips to keep in mind as you establish your routines:

- Be realistic.

- Honor the season you're in.

- Incorporate getting outside in daylight into your morning routine.

- Whenever possible, reduce screen time and exposure to blue/bright lights in the evening hours.

My morning and evening routines change regularly based on my season of life. This is not something to be strict or rigid about; I have found that I need different things depending on my circumstances and the needs of my family. Staying flexible is key to consistency.

If it sounds intimidating to create new routines, remember some of the reframes we discussed in chapter 1. Avoid the all-or-nothing mentality, choose grace over guilt when things don't go as planned, and remember that every little bit counts.

> Staying flexible is key to consistency.

Perfection is not required to experience benefits. You can set up realistic, practical routines in your day-to-day life that will support your body's natural rhythms.

Reconnect with Nature

Years ago, we had to work hard to find devices (remember computer labs and pay phones?). These days, the script has flipped. Now we have to be intentional about unplugging and getting outside, or it's unlikely to happen. Spending time in nature has a direct positive impact on our health and well-being.

Sample Routines

As you think through creating your own routines, here are a few examples you might be able to incorporate into your unique season of life.

Short Morning Routine

- Wake up and drink water.
- Shower.
- Get dressed.
- Make the bed and open the curtains.
- Spend 10–15 minutes journaling/praying/doing Pilates (you can rotate these habits throughout the week).
- Eat breakfast and step outside to get morning sunlight on your eyes.

Leisurely Morning Routine

- Wake up and drink water.
- Make the bed and open the curtains.
- Brew coffee/tea while making a nourishing breakfast.
- Enjoy breakfast and coffee/tea outside when possible to get sunlight on your eyes.
- Journal/pray/make a gratitude list.
- Exercise.
- Shower.
- Listen to an inspirational or educational podcast while getting ready for the day.

Here are some of the benefits of regularly spending time in green spaces[11]:

- reduction in anxiety, stress, and depression

- increased immune health and brain function

- improved personal relationships, creativity, and overall well-being

Short Evening Routine

- Sunset: switch screens to evening mode (you can adjust this setting on your phone and your computer).
- One hour before bed: wrap up screen time on computer, phone, and TV.
- Wash face and brush teeth.
- Read in bed before falling asleep (bonus: use red-tinted light bulbs in the bedroom to reduce exposure to bright lights and promote the release of melatonin).

Leisurely Evening Routine

- Sunset: switch screens to evening mode (you can adjust this setting on your phone and your computer).
- After dark: wear blue light–blocking glasses to reduce exposure to bright lights.
- One hour before bed: wrap up screen time on computer, phone, and TV.
- Take a relaxing bath in dim lighting (add Epsom salts or essential oils to increase relaxation).
- Wash face and brush teeth.
- Read in bed before falling asleep (bonus: use red-tinted light bulbs in the bedroom to reduce exposure to bright lights and promote the release of melatonin).

There are numerous health benefits from spending time in the great outdoors. Vitamin D from safe sun exposure supports the absorption of calcium, leading to better bone health,[12] and strengthens the immune system so your body is better able to fight off illness and infection.[13] Exposure to naturally occurring bacteria in dirt and soil can increase the beneficial bacteria in your intestinal tract, which is good for gut health.[14] Improved gut health has been linked to better digestion, increased absorption of nutrients, a stronger immune system, and improved mood and mental health.[15] That's why when my kids ask to play in the dirt, I (almost) always say yes!

If your schedule is already full, it may feel daunting to try to add spending time in nature. Here are some practical ideas, no matter where you live:

Step outside more often. Taking your lunch to a park or going for a walk in a neighborhood park is an easy way to get outside and connect with nature, even if you only have ten minutes. If you use public transportation, you might consider getting off at an earlier stop and walking the rest of the way. If you use a car, you might want to park in the farthest spot at the grocery store or arrive at an appointment early and walk around for a few minutes beforehand.

Plant a garden. Planting a garden can be a relaxing way to unplug and enjoy nature. If you live in a small space, try a vertical garden or start with a few potted herbs and plants.

Take your workout outdoors! Roll out your mat outside, where you have room to stretch, breathe in fresh air, and feel the breeze on your skin. Or go for a long walk, device-free. Exercising in nature is a wonderful way to care for your health and reap the benefits of movement, sunshine, and fresh air in an energizing, efficient way.

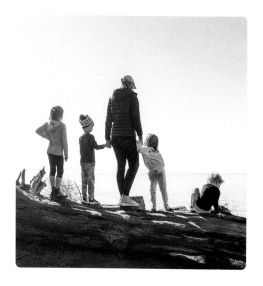

Spend time near trees. The practice of forest bathing is becoming more popular as research shows that spending time in a forest can have a positive effect on mood, stress, blood pressure, focus, and the immune system.[16] Forest bathing is essentially immersing yourself in nature and practicing mindfulness to calm the nervous system. Even if you don't live near a forest, you can go for a hike or a walk to reap the benefits of connecting with nature and unplugging all at the same time.

Practice grounding. Grounding, also known as earthing, is the act of walking barefoot or sitting on the ground outdoors. Growing research indicates it can have a positive impact on our health, as it improves sleep and reduces pain. While this might sound a little "woo-woo" at first, scientific studies have shown that as modern living disconnects us from nature, the simple act of taking off our shoes and walking barefoot outside can have a direct physiological effect on our bodies—reducing inflammation, improving heart rate variability, and fighting chronic stress, among other benefits.[17]

The goal of unplugging is not to live a life without technology but simply to create a healthy, balanced relationship with screens. When we take time to disconnect from our devices, we create space for our minds and our bodies to flourish.

 ## Put It into Practice

- **Try a digital detox** to reset your relationship with technology. (See the sidebar at the end of this chapter to choose a detox that suits your needs and goals.)

- **Step outside** in the morning. Even five minutes outside can be beneficial to your health.

- **Adjust the screen settings** on your computer and phone to activate "night mode" in the evening.

- **Invest in a pair** of blue light–blocking glasses.

- **Swap out your bedside light** for a bulb with a red glow to support melatonin production and to prepare your mind and body for a night of deep, restful sleep.

Digital Detox

Spending intentional time away from screens can be helpful in restoring balance to our relationship with technology. If you're looking to create healthier screen boundaries, here are a few options for a digital detox, whether you want to make a small change or do an overhaul.

Reduce—Level 1

If you're hoping to reduce your screen time, you might consider this option. Give your devices a bedtime and a wake-up time. Each evening at a designated time (at least one hour before you go to bed), plug your devices into their charging station (not in the bedroom) and turn off the TV. Similarly, designate a time that you'll use your devices again in the morning. This will help you bookend your day with intentional screen-free time to support a healthy, balanced relationship with technology.

Reset—Level 2

If you're feeling too plugged in to your technology, you may need a reset. For two days, remove your favorite (and most addicting) apps from your phone. Notice when you want to start scrolling out of habit, and in those moments, choose to be present with those around you or open a book instead. Ask for accountability from someone you trust to help you stick to your goal. Notice how you feel after two days of reduced phone use. Repeat this challenge as often as needed, perhaps even implementing it as a weekend routine.

Detox—Level 3

If technology is starting to interfere with the way you feel each day and the way you interact with those around you, you might be ready for more drastic action. Remove your favorite (and most addicting) apps from your phone for a longer period—perhaps one week or one month. In addition, set a bedtime and a wake-up time for all devices (including TV). Be intentional about not replacing one app with another, or one form of technology with another. Throughout your detox, journal about how you feel and what you want to continue when your detox is complete.

connect

When the *i* is replaced with *we*, even illness becomes wellness.

Unknown

When the twins entered our family, our entire world changed. Between feedings, naps, diaper changes, doctor appointments, snacks, potty training, school drop-offs, and caring for our three- and five-year-old, our days felt incredibly full. Add working from home to the mix, and doing anything beyond our regular routine felt nearly impossible. During this chaotic season, there was one thing we clung to as our primary method of survival: our daily routine.

Friends would invite me to meet up for playdates, go for a walk, or come over for dinner. When the phone would buzz, I'd have an internal debate over

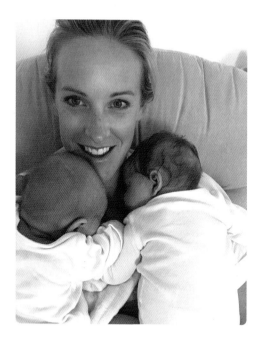

whether it was worth it to skip naps, delay feedings, fall behind on my work, and forgo dinner prep, all so I could say yes to seeing a friend. After I weighed all the factors, nine times out of ten my answer was "I'm sorry—I can't."

After a few months of rarely being available, the invitations started to dwindle. I understood why—when someone says no nearly every time you ask, it doesn't exactly encourage you to keep reaching out. As a result, my circle of friends began to shrink. When the pandemic hit a few months later, my social network took another major hit. The larger community of people we once saw at church, at the park, or at school all disappeared. When we were stuck at home and our community was stripped away, I realized just how much a smile from another mom or a quick hug from a friend contributes to an overall feeling of life satisfaction. While there were benefits to stripping away some of the nonessentials and focusing on the relationships closest to me (hello, stay-at-home orders), I felt lonely.

And loneliness isn't confined just to pandemic times. We can feel disconnected at all stages of life, whether we're living alone or surrounded by other people.

The Value of Community

Over the past few years, loneliness has been on the rise.[1] As we gain an awareness of this trend, we have an opportunity to reconsider and reevaluate our social connections, our relationships, and our community.

We inhabit a world that looks considerably different from the one generations before us lived in. Many of us don't live near extended family, and our schedules move at an unrelenting pace. As a result, it can be hard to regularly spend time with friends and family. We juggle work, travel, volunteering, sporting events, carpooling, errands, and more. Sometimes spending time with others just seems too complicated to arrange, so it takes a back seat. While it's true that we can stay connected with people through technology, nothing can compare to the value of in-person relationships. We can even have anything delivered to our door with the click of a button, removing all social interaction in the process.

You may also be in a season that makes it hard to feel connected to others the way you'd like. Perhaps you're in a phase of nonstop caretaking, as I was after my twins were born. Or you may be battling an illness that makes it hard to participate in social events. Perhaps your current work schedule offers little margin for gathering with friends, or maybe you're so tapped out by the end of the day that making plans requires more energy than you can muster.

With all these factors, it's easy to see why we're at risk for isolation and loneliness.

According to the latest research, age, gender, and culture all play a factor in our social connections, as well as how lonely we may feel.[2] Our experience of community may also be influenced by whether we were raised in (or live in) an individualistic culture or a collectivist culture. Individualistic cultures value self-reliance and have loose social networks. These cultures are heavily influenced by "chosen relationships." Collectivist cultures, in contrast, encourage interdependence.

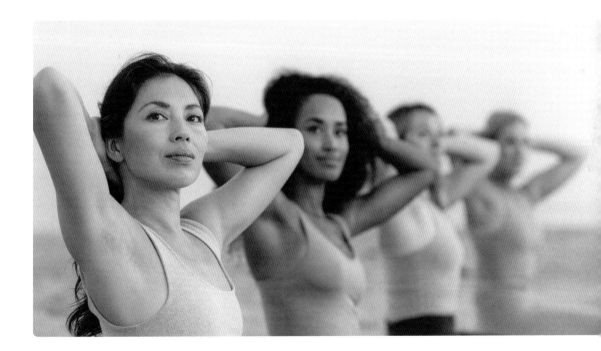

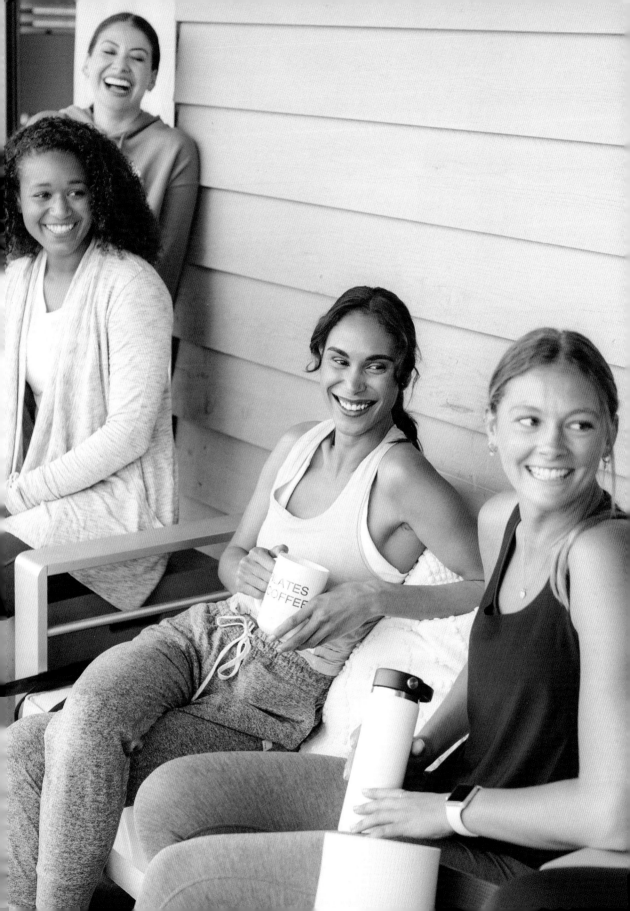

Connection is a basic human need—
we were designed to be
in relationship with others.

They are characterized by tightly knit social networks and dominated by extended family and members of the group.[3] What this means for those of us in individualistic Western cultures is that we must be more intentional about the ways we create community and connection with others.

Connection is a basic human need—we were designed to be in relationship with others. Just as we need water, air, and food, we need one another. Positive social connections have been shown to have the following benefits:

- improved immune health

- lower blood pressure

- increased ability to recover from disease

- reduced levels of anxiety and depression

- increased longevity

The flip side is also true. A lack of social connection has been associated with the following harmful effects:

- increased risk of death

- increased risk of cardiovascular disease, atherosclerosis, high blood pressure, and cancer

- slower wound healing

- delayed cancer recovery

- impaired immune function and increased inflammatory biomarkers[4]

If we're not making human connection a priority, we're missing out on a significant part of what it means to be well. Human connection matters a lot—for the mind and for the body.

Creating Community and Deepening Connections

There are many ways to create positive social connections—there's no one-size-fits-all formula for everyone, and our relationships may look different in different seasons. But whatever it looks like for you right now, developing positive relationships is a vital investment in your health. Just as we schedule workouts or plan meals for the week, it's equally important to consider how we can strengthen our relationships.

Maybe as you take stock of your life right now, you recognize that this is an area you want to grow in. If so, it may be tempting to think you need to go out and make a bunch of new friends. But it doesn't have to be that complicated. You can start by looking at the connections you already have.

What relationships are most important to you? This may seem obvious, but the loudest voices are not always the ones we value most. If we aren't intentional with our time, we will end up giving our attention to lesser priorities.

My marriage is one of the relationships I want to invest in most. In some seasons that has meant going to counseling together to get on the same page, improve communication, and process complicated situations. In other seasons it has meant arranging for a babysitter to watch the kids so we could go on weekly or monthly date nights. And in some cases, it has meant going to great lengths to arrange childcare and clear our schedules so we could go on a trip, just the two of us—a monumental feat during this season, but one that is always worth it for the sake of our marriage. If you aren't married, think of a focal relationship in your life that you want to make sure you're pouring into. It might be with a parent, grandparent, sibling, or close friend—the key is to take a moment to think about the relationships that matter most and take intentional action to foster a sense of connection.

I greatly value my friendships. But who knew friendship could be so complicated? It was a challenging transition for me to go from having best friends in college to making new friendships as an adult. When I was in college, my friends were everything to me—they were the people I had meals with, worked out with, went shopping with, confided in, laughed with, and lived with.

When I entered the post-college world of adulthood, got married, and moved to a new city, I found myself looking for local friends who could fill all those needs and check all the boxes—and it wasn't happening. I met new and interesting acquaintances, but I felt like I just couldn't find "my people."

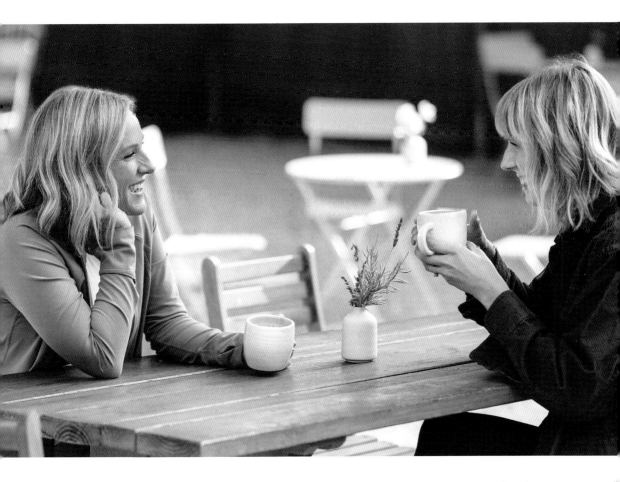

Over time, I realized I was going about relationships all wrong. I was looking for one person who could be everything my college friends were to me. So I made a mindset shift that allowed me to appreciate my new friendships in a different way. I stopped looking for one best friend and started appreciating the unique things about each person I met.

Maybe you have a solid group of friends, and you already feel filled up in this area. Or you may feel like I did—that you still haven't found your people. If you're waiting for that one perfect best friend, it might help to shift your approach to allow different people to fill different needs. For example, you may have one friend you can talk to for hours about anything, big or small. You may have another friend who is a great walking partner—someone you enjoy spending time with, but you may not pour out your heart to them. When we take the pressure off people to be

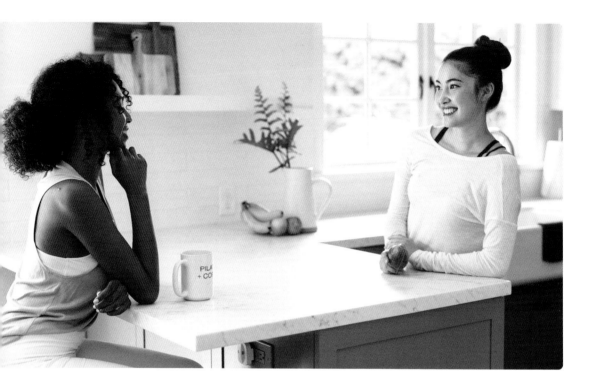

all things to us, it frees us up to appreciate the community we have and reap the health benefits of positive, life-giving connections.

If you don't know where to start in cultivating new friendships and improving the relationships you have, start small. As with the other areas we've discussed, it doesn't have to be all or nothing, and it doesn't have to be overwhelming.

When I was feeling unfulfilled in my friendships, I realized I was expecting meaningful community to magically appear, with little effort on my part. But that wasn't happening, so I had to change my approach. I needed to take the first step. Instead of waiting for invitations to come to me, I chose to be the initiator.

This can be nerve wracking—you may feel insecure, wondering if the person you invited will say yes or reciprocate. But most people are longing for connection too, and they will be blessed by your willingness to reach out. And if they say no, remember that nine times out of ten, it's not personal!

So here's my challenge to you (and me): make the first move. Instead of hoping community will find you, create it yourself. Instead of waiting for a friend to reach out to you, reach out to them first. Send a text or a funny meme when you see something that reminds you of them. Invite them to join you for a morning walk or a Pilates class.

Another way to build connection is to offer help . . . or to ask for help. If you make a big batch of soup that you may not be able to finish on your own, offer to drop some off on a friend's doorstep. If you're running to the farmers market, text a friend to see if you can pick anything up for them. If you're willing to be a little vulnerable (which is proven to enhance relationships[6]), ask for advice or help when you need it.

If vulnerability seems scary at first, you can ease into that space by asking for a restaurant recommendation. Then you can take it to the next level by asking a friend if you can borrow something or if they'd be able to run an errand for you when you're sick or in a bind. The truth is, most people will be honored to be asked.

So, reach out. Text a friend. Invite a family over for dinner. Join an online community. Seek out the type of people you want to surround yourself with, and make the first move. Your health (and happiness) depends on it.

Relationship Inventory

Make a list of the primary relationships in your life—the people you interact with on a daily or weekly basis. These are the people you live with, work with, meet up with, and share your life with. The list doesn't need to be long to be valuable. Once you've made your list, circle two or three relationships you'd like to be intentional about developing.

Now write down ways you can invest in each relationship you circled. This may look like making plans with a friend to meet for coffee, scheduling a date night with your spouse, or carving out one-on-one time with a child. It could also look like having a hard conversation, setting a new boundary, or meeting with a therapist.

As you look at the list of relationships above, is there an area of your life where you would benefit from having more support (e.g., wellness, career, motherhood, or grief)? Are there certain social connections that are currently bringing you down? Is there anything you can do to set boundaries or seek help in this area?

Surround Yourself with Support

Years ago, when I did one-on-one health coaching for my Pilates clients, I noticed a common struggle for women I worked with. Many of them felt unsupported by their family and friends when it came to their wellness goals.

One client was ready to feel good again after years of not feeling well and putting her health on the back burner. She wanted to build strength, take control of her back pain, and cook more nourishing foods for herself and her family instead of relying on takeout each night. Beyond that, she wanted to repair her relationship with her body. For as long as she could remember, she'd been unhappy with the size and shape of her body.

But she was struggling because her husband and her mother didn't understand her desire to make healthy changes. Even though her mother would remind her that she hadn't lost the baby weight yet, the negative comments only increased as my client began to make healthy changes. My client's husband was also resistant to the change. He liked their nightly takeout routine and complained when she made a new healthy recipe. He was less than enthusiastic about watching the kids on the weekends so she could go to her Pilates class.

It can be a challenge to feel unsupported on our wellness journey. The truth is, when you decide to make a change to improve your health, others are not always excited. Sometimes they don't take it seriously, sometimes they make disparaging comments, and sometimes they even feel threatened by your progress.

This is one of the reasons I created an online community. I saw a huge need for women to find support and encouragement on their journey toward becoming the healthiest version of themselves. This work is hard to do alone—and it's even harder when it feels like others are against you. I wanted a space where women know they're not alone, and where they're fully supported and celebrated for the positive changes they're making. This unwavering, nonjudgmental support can be a game changer in our ability to shift our habits and routines to support our wholeness.

If you find that key people in your life aren't on board with your health and wellness goals, here a few tips to help you as you communicate with them:

Share your why. Instead of launching into a lecture about why exercise or healthy eating is important, share what led you to make this change. Did you find a workout routine that sparked enjoyment instead of dread? Did you feel

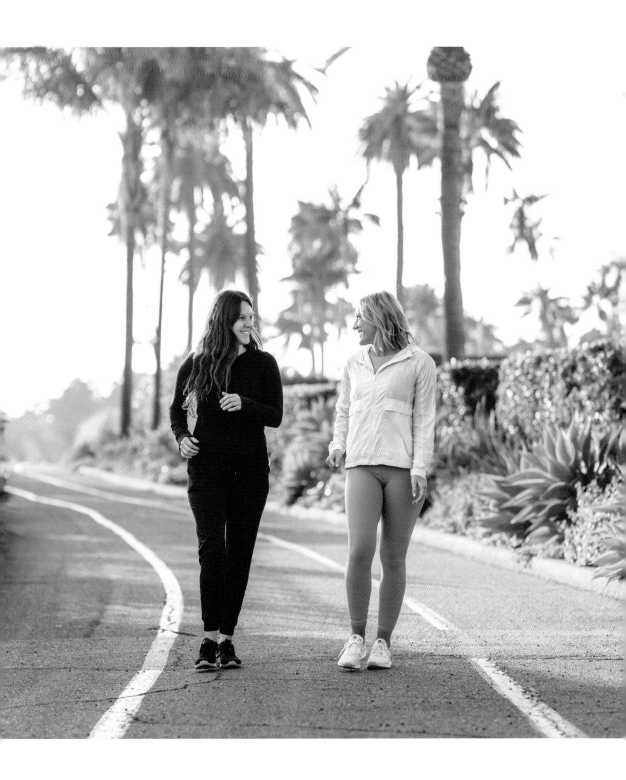

dissatisfied with the way you were feeling? Are you craving more energy in your day-to-day activities? Are you committed to aging well? Letting people in on your journey will help them understand that you need support and that this change is about you, not them.

Be open about your struggles, and ask for support. Sometimes friends and family assume you're trying to be better than they are because you're no longer eating the same foods or participating in the same activities (such as binge drinking on the weekend, eating ice cream on the couch every night, or scrolling on your phone for hours). When you're open about how challenging it is to replace old habits and when you ask for support, you give them an opportunity to participate in the journey with you.

Also, be as specific as possible about the kind of support you need. Maybe you just want your spouse to be open to trying some new recipes. Or maybe you'd love for your friend to join you for a morning walk. Or maybe you'd rather not be the center of attention when you pass on a second drink. Whatever support you need, speak up so those around you can be a part of your quest for well-being.

> ## Cultivating positive relationships is a lifelong endeavor.

Remember that it's probably not about you. When we make healthy changes, it can make other people uncomfortable. If others make negative comments or show a lack of support, it's probably more about them and less about you. Keep this in mind, and try to be gentle with them. Some people may come around eventually. Others may not—and that's okay. As you set out on this journey to embrace a new approach to wellness, it helps to surround yourself with a like-minded community so you'll stay grounded in what matters most to you. I've tried to surround myself with people who value true wellness and who understand that progress is more important than perfection—people who understand that there are much more interesting things to talk about than the way we look! Surrounding yourself with supportive, like-minded friends will make it easier—and more fun—to create lasting changes on your health and wellness journey.

Cultivating positive relationships is a lifelong endeavor. Just as your exercise routine will look different in various seasons of life, the same is true with relationships. It took me a while to recognize my need for more support and friendship after the twins were born. For the first few years, I was so busy changing diapers, cleaning up messes, preparing meals, and trying to stay connected to my husband that I didn't have the bandwidth to reach beyond the relationships within my own home.

Little by little, as our routines shifted and my capacity increased, I was able to make small investments into relationships that I hadn't been showing up for and cultivate new ones. By making the first move, stepping into uncomfortable situations, and being vulnerable, I've found that my life satisfaction has improved along with my relationships. This takes ongoing intentionality on my part, and I still have room to grow in this area. But my life is richer for the effort.

Put It into Practice

- **Text or call one friend** each day just to check in and connect.

- **Meet up with a friend or family member** for a weekly walk. You'll reap the benefits of social connection, exercise, and being outdoors, all in one efficient meetup.

- **Make the first move:** invite a friend to meet for coffee, or ask a new friend for a local recommendation to spark connection and open the door for friendship.

- **Join a group or an organization** that supports your values where you can find like-minded people.

- **Join an online community** to support you in an area where you need it. (Might I suggest the Lindywell community? We're here for you!)

- **When you're standing in line** at the grocery store, look up, smile, say hello, make small talk, and notice how the personal connection makes you feel.

From the Lindywell Community
Joan J.

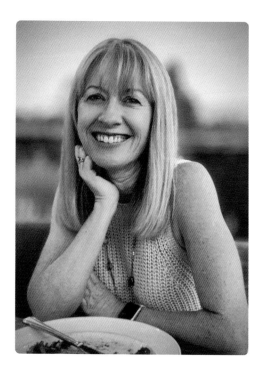

I live in beautiful Moorpark, California. I start my days early to have time to read the Bible, stretch, do Pilates, text a friend, and walk the dog before I begin my work as a film and TV scriptwriter. As a widow of five years, I'm thankful for my extended family, my church, and my hobbies that allow me to stay connected to others.

Many of the physical challenges I've faced stem from stress and anxiety. When my husband was dying, I found myself dry heaving each morning—a response to stress. I've also struggled with migraines, tight muscles, and teeth grinding, which are also rooted in my anxiety.

I've gone to therapy to get to what's underneath my stress and to learn healthier ways to deal with it—breathing, praying, exercising, making a mental gratitude list, getting fresh air, or doing the next right thing (which can be as small as brushing my teeth).

I can get overwhelmed when interacting with large groups. At the same time, I need love, and I enjoy human connection and community. So I'm very intentional, particularly in this stage of my life, about carving out family time and creating interaction with others. ·

I love to read and discuss what I'm learning, so a number of years ago, I invited a handful of women—some I knew pretty well and some I wanted to get to know better—to start a weekly wine and Bible study group. Over the years, we've laughed uncontrollably, cried deeply, and held one another up. We've walked together through life's great joys (weddings, career successes, and the births of grand-children) and great sorrows (betrayals, loss of employment, and the deaths of spouses and parents).

We've traveled together and met online when we couldn't meet in person, and every Christmas we gather at my house for my "I Cook Once a Year" dinner. Despite my lack of practice, the food almost always turns out, and the company makes it a win no matter what happens. We go around the table, sharing our reflections from the past year and our hopes for the year to come.

As I once heard someone say, "My head is a dangerous place; I shouldn't go there alone!" In this community, we help one another get out of our heads by sharing what's in them—our doubts, fears, and negative thoughts—and by speaking truth, love, and kindness to one another as well as sharing what has worked for us. (We share the names of doctors, therapists, and home-repair workers too!)

I had to be intentional, take a chance, and reach out to surround myself with community. But as intimidating as it seemed at first, these relationships have brought richness and meaning to my life.

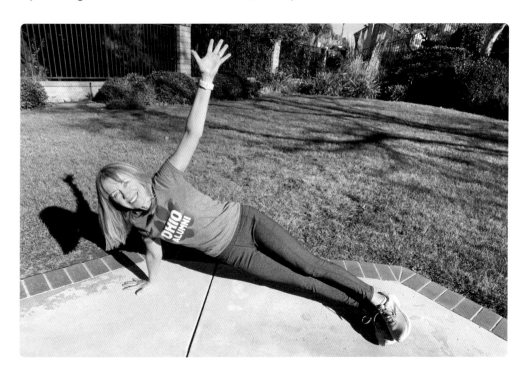

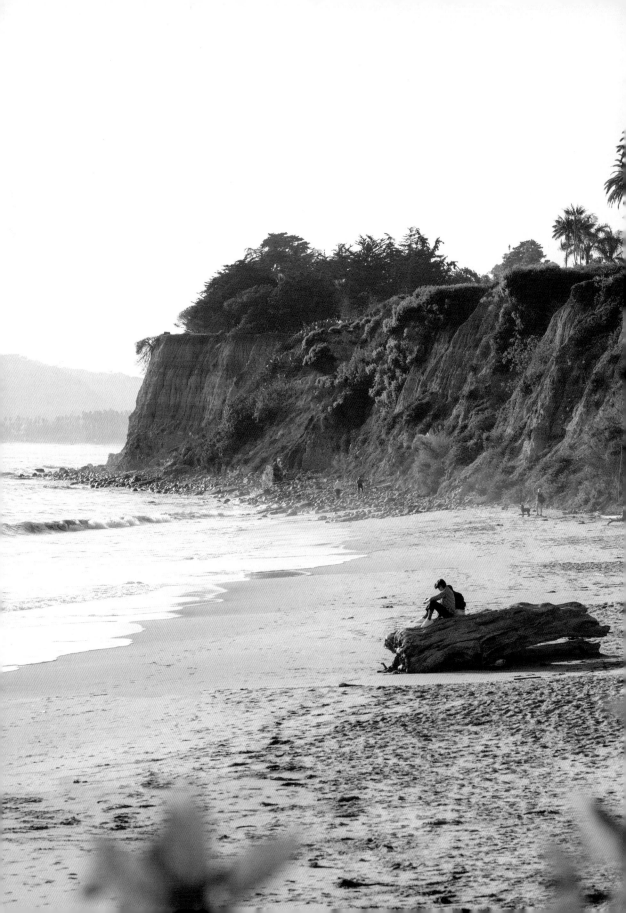

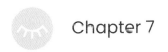

Chapter 7

rest

When you rest, you catch your breath, and it fills your lungs and holds you up, like water wings.

Anne Lamott

If your life is anything like mine, items are added to your to-do list faster than you can check them off, and it feels like you can never get ahead. On any given day, my texts go unanswered, my inbox overflows, the dishes pile up, and the laundry is in constant need of folding. The world moves quickly, and it takes a lot of work to keep up (on the rare days we can!). As a result, we operate at a pace that is largely unsustainable. I would go so far as to say that as a culture—and specifically for women—we are in the early stages of an epidemic of burnout.

Unfortunately, I speak from experience.

When I received my health diagnosis a few years ago, I was caught off guard. Lab results revealed that my hormones were completely out of balance.

As I sat in my doctor's office to review my results, she told me I had many risk factors for autoimmune disease. While the test results revealed that an auto-immune disease was not currently present, she told me that I absolutely had to make changes. Thankfully, there were steps I could take to improve my health, but it would take time, intentionality, and perhaps most important of all, more rest.

The go-go-go lifestyle has become
the norm in our society,
but it's only a matter of time
before we crash.

As a working mom of four, I found the instruction to slow down and rest to be one of the most challenging assignments I could receive. Just that morning, I'd been woken before dawn by a toddler who had escaped his crib, squealed with excitement, and decided it was time for the rest of the house to wake up too. The day continued at breakneck speed while I did my best to keep up, just like I'd done the day before.

Not only was rest a logistical challenge in my season of life, it was also not in my nature. As someone who is prone to taking action to try to gain a sense of control, I would have preferred a to-do list from my doctor—something I could get started on right away.

As I sat in her office, she said to me, "Robin, I see that you are a very capable woman. You can handle a lot, but you don't know when to say that enough is enough. Your body is telling you that you need to slow down. And while there are practical things you can do, like take supplements and add healing foods, the number one thing you need to do is do *less*."

Essentially, I was living in a state of fight or flight. Without my even realizing it, this way of living had become my new normal. My nervous system was always on high alert, and I rarely had a chance to rest, recover, and reset. (The mere noise level in my house prompted my body to respond as if there were a threat behind every corner.) My body and my brain were helping me function—they stayed on overdrive to help me meet the demands of my job, my home, and my relationships. But I couldn't keep up that pace forever.

I was operating in a state of disconnection from my body. Although I was receiving warning signs, I just kept powering through. As my test results revealed, my body was entering a state of burnout. Around the same time, I began hearing from friend after friend that they, too, were in a similar situation: experiencing feelings of exhaustion, low sex drive, unexplained weight gain, hair loss, muscle aches, and digestive issues.

What I came to understand was that rest is important for my health, regardless of an official diagnosis. It's essential for all of us, at every stage of life. The go-go-go lifestyle has become the norm in our society, but it's only a matter of time before we crash . . . unless we do something about it.

My experience was a wake-up call for me. Not only did my ego take a hit (I mean, I teach this for a living!), but I also discovered that my approach to wellness at the time was incomplete. While I was listening to my body, exercising, preparing nourishing meals, and drinking plenty of water, I was pushing too hard when what my body really needed was to slow down. Since discovering this imbalance, I've spoken with countless women in similar situations. If you're in a state of constant motion, with little space for rest, I have a hunch this way of life is taking a toll on you, too.

So what does it truly mean to rest? Rest can look like a good night of sleep, but it goes much deeper than that. Part of resting is considering our rhythms throughout the days, weeks, and years as well. We need both sleep and healthy rhythms to support the regeneration of our minds and bodies. When we get this kind of rest, we'll feel our best, day in and day out.

Improving Your Quality of Sleep

I'm guessing you already know how important sleep is, but it's worth noting just what an impact it has on the body. Quality sleep can have the following benefits:

- improved immune response

- reduced risk of disease

- increased brain performance

- improved mood

- decreased stress[1]

It's during sleep that our brains rejuvenate and our bodies recover. Biological processes that ward off diseases such as dementia and Alzheimer's take place while we're sleeping.[2] Our brains synthesize information and remove toxins that are damaging to our mental and physical health when we are asleep. Lack of sleep has been linked to weight fluctuations, increased cravings, insulin resistance, depression, and anxiety.[3]

Getting enough sleep has a significant impact on every area of life. Even appetite and metabolism are impacted by the quality of our sleep.[4] When I have a poor night of sleep, I know my cravings will be elevated the following day. I wake up craving starchy breakfast foods such as bagels, muffins, and scones—anything to give me a quick boost of serotonin. I drink more coffee, and in the afternoon I reach for sweets to keep me going. The cycle continues until my head hits the pillow at night. Beyond the cravings, my mood is off, my energy is low, and my cognitive processes feel foggy and slow. But when I get a good night of sleep, I feel more balanced and in control of how I feel and act.

Perhaps you agree that sleep is important, but you're in a season when good sleep just doesn't seem possible. Maybe you're in a stressful work situation or you're working the night shift or you have several jobs to make ends meet. Maybe you have a child who doesn't sleep through the night, or your insomnia feels completely out of your control. Stages of life and hormonal changes can have a direct impact on the quality of your sleep. If you're struggling in this area, it's okay. Take a deep breath and relax your shoulders. The goal is not to add more stress to your plate but to empower you to start where you are, work with what you have, and give yourself plenty of grace along the way.

When it comes to wellness, sleep is just as important as exercising and nutrition. So let's get practical. How can we set ourselves up for success in this area? Here are a few research-backed tips and strategies for getting the best night of sleep possible:

- **Step outside** to get daylight on your eyes each morning before ten o'clock (see chapter 5 for more details).

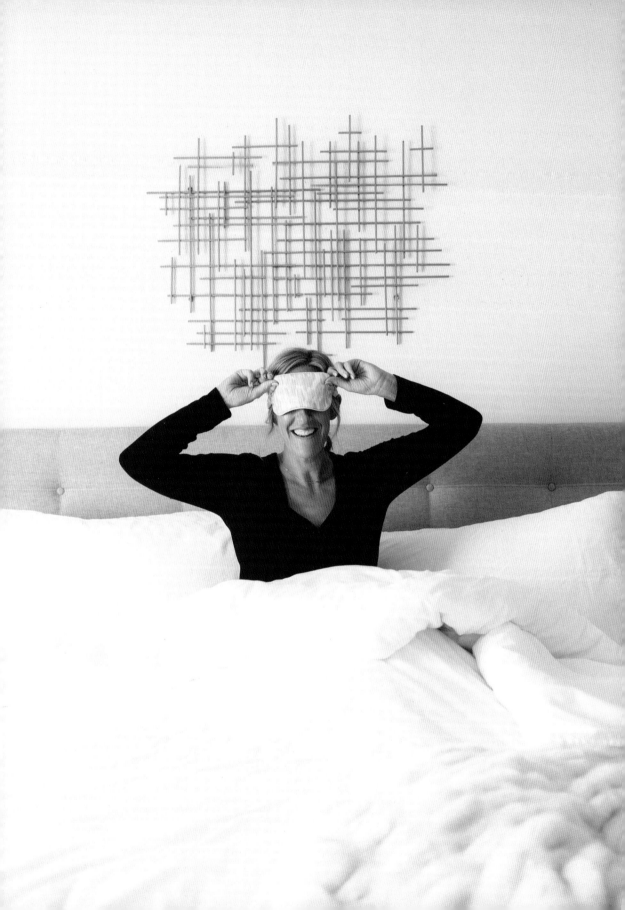

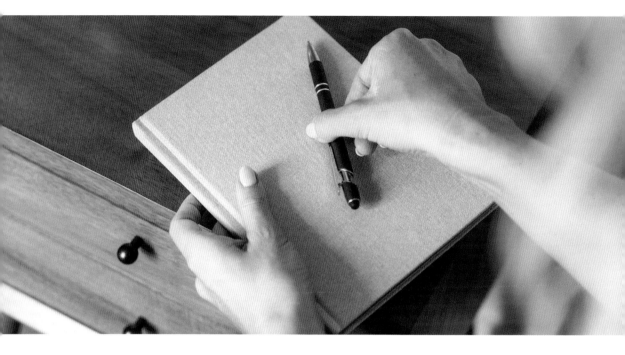

- **Add movement** into your day. Exercise has been shown to improve sleep.[5]

- **Unplug from electronic devices** at least one hour before bed. (If possible, invest in a pair of blue light–blocking glasses to wear when looking at screens after dark.) Consider replacing evening screen time with an old-fashioned book.

- **Keep a notepad by your bed** to jot down any lingering thoughts that are running around in your head. This will provide a way to slow your thoughts and prepare you for sleep.

- **Swap out traditional bedroom light bulbs** for red-hued lights to promote better sleep. (For those who wake up often in the night, red lights have been shown to keep the body in a more relaxed state compared to blue-tone lights, which tell the brain it's time to wake up.[6] I like to use salt lamps when I wake up at night.)

- **Invest in black-out shades or a comfortable sleep mask** to block out light. Even the smallest bit of light shining in a room at night has been shown to disrupt deep sleep.[7]

- **Relax or read in a warm bath** with Epsom salts to calm the body and relieve stress.

- **Charge your phone in another room.** Out of sight, out of mind—and, most important, out of reach.

If deep sleep still eludes you, here are a few additional tips that might help:

- **Practice deep breathing** while lying in bed.

- **Before you climb into bed,** spend ten minutes stretching and breathing on your mat to help your body release tension and allow your mind to unwind (see relaxation exercise at the end of this chapter).

A Balance of Movement and Rest

When crafting a Pilates workout for my clients, I structure the routine so there's a balance between movement and rest. We spend most of our time in motion on the mat: performing exercises, flowing through movements, and challenging our bodies to strengthen and stretch. But there are also intentional moments of rest. These moments of rest come when our bodies need it most—perhaps after a challenging series of exercises or at the beginning and the end of the workout to allow for a transition onto and off the mat.

Similarly, in a strenuous workout such as weight lifting, the rest day after an intense session is not a luxury; it's essential so muscles can repair and recover. Both the challenging days and the days of rest are necessary to get results.

In the same way, we need a balance between movement and rest in our lives. This applies at all levels—annually, seasonally, monthly, weekly, and daily. We aren't designed to live in a state of constant doing, yet that's how many of us spend our time. It wasn't until I was faced with my own limitations that I was forced to take a hard look at my habits and rhythms.

I was already pretty intentional about this—I unplugged from work on the weekends and even stopped working at night to help me recharge. I made it a point to get quality sleep at night (a feat in itself with young kids in the house). I prided myself on having good work/life boundaries. I took time to do things that filled my cup. But I didn't have a plan in place for prioritizing true rest throughout the week.

I like to be in motion. One of the ways I de-stress is to declutter. I enjoy cultivating a beautiful home, so I organize, fold laundry, freshen up, and decorate. I sort my kids' clothes and donate items they've grown out of. I run to Target, I meal prep for the week ahead, and I go on hikes, walks, and other adventures. These things are all good and life giving for me, but none of those activities qualify as true rest for my body and mind.

Your hobbies and habits may be different from mine. Perhaps you love to travel, cook, ride horses, or spend time with friends. Perhaps you enjoy volunteering, leading community groups, serving on a board, or supporting your local church. (Or maybe you don't have the time or energy for hobbies at all right now!) But just as our bodies need movement, connection, and nourishment, they also need rest.

Implementing Rhythms of Rest

Apart from sleep, how do you currently rest?

I posed this question to a few friends recently, and while they reported plenty of things they like to do in their downtime, few had a solid answer for how they make time and space to rest their minds and bodies.

We tend to think of rest as a luxury or even a guilty pleasure. Or, depending on how you were brought up, you might even view it as lazy. But rest isn't something

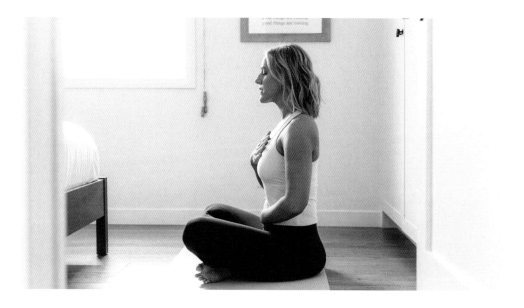

to be enjoyed only after all our work is finished; it's actually a necessary part of a balanced life. Rest has been shown to improve health in the following ways:

- reducing stress

- sparking creativity

- boosting immune health[8]

- promoting healthy hormonal balance[9]

- slowing the aging process[10]

- improving brain function[11]

- increasing productivity (this sounds counterintuitive, I know!)[12]

Even if we know rest is important, it's easy for guilt to creep in. You may associate rest with being lazy or unproductive. Or perhaps you were criticized for resting as a child, and you live with the subconscious feeling that someone is watching over your shoulder and there's no time for rest. Maybe you're a caregiver and you worry that any time you take for yourself is selfish.

I've battled feelings of guilt when it comes to rest too. If I take time for myself, that usually means someone else is taking more of the load, whether that's Matt, a work colleague, or a friend. I feel bad for choosing rest instead of doing something that feels productive, playing with my kids, or meeting up with friends. As a result, it's tempting to put rest on the back burner for when I have time. But I'm learning that rest is not a form of indulgence, and it doesn't equate to idleness. Rather, it's essential to good health. If we don't create space for rest, we will end up burning out or experiencing health issues. I speak from experience, and I want to help you avoid the mistakes I've made.

Learning to rest requires that we listen to and honor our bodies' needs. If you find yourself getting sick frequently, you likely need more rest. If you're regularly exhausted, you likely need more rest. If you push yourself to your limits most days, you need more rest. You can start simply by noticing your body's cues, and then try to find practical ways you can honor that need for rest.

For example, when you're feeling worn down, you may choose to cancel your afternoon plans and take a nap instead. Or rather than using your five minutes of

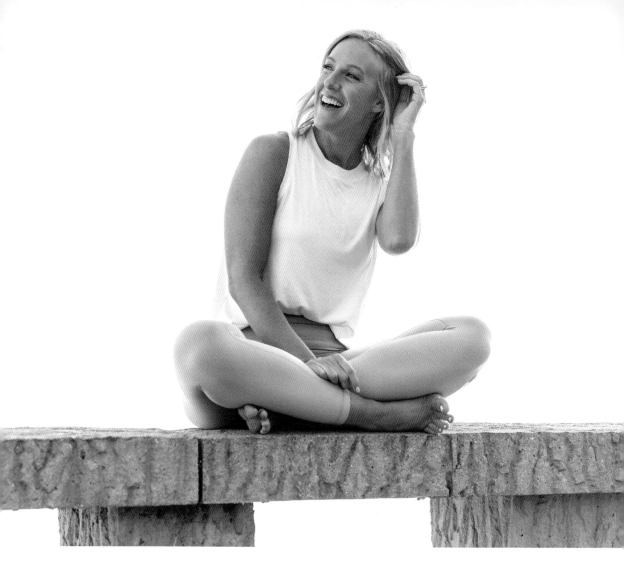

downtime before your next appointment to scroll social media (further stimulating your brain), you can lie on your back, close your eyes, and take a few deep breaths.

As with scheduling workouts and planning meals, incorporating rhythms of rest requires intentionality. I've found that the best way to ensure true rest is to schedule it into weekly, monthly, and annual rhythms.

Weekly Rhythms of Rest

On a weekly basis, you might experiment with honoring the Sabbath (a day of rest from all work). Many people choose to do this on Saturday or Sunday, but feel free to choose any day that works with your schedule. Or you might schedule a few hours of rest on a specific day, just as you'd schedule a coffee date with a friend or a doctor appointment. During this scheduled time, try to find something that allows you to truly slow down, quiet the noise from the outside world, and rejuvenate your mind and body. You could take a nap, sit outside in the shade, or read a book while lounging on the couch in your coziest clothes. You could make it a point to actually take your lunch break and sit on a bench at a park. If your budget allows, you could schedule a massage, a facial, a manicure, or a hair appointment, if that's something that truly helps you slow down and doesn't feel like something else to cross off your to-do list. (And make sure you put down your phone and rest during this time!)

Monthly Rhythms of Rest

On a monthly basis, you can look at your calendar and designate weekends of rest to counterbalance all your other commitments and activities. As a family, if we have too many overscheduled weekends in a row (even if they're fun!), we feel the effects. We need a balance of rest and activity in the flow of our month to function best. Slow mornings at home are good for the soul (and the nervous system).

Annual Rhythms of Rest

On an annual basis, consider implementing rejuvenation weeks. This involves taking time out of your ordinary responsibilities at work and at home, whether you go somewhere or stay at home. While it can be difficult to slow down our pace and to plan all the logistics to make this happen, it's something we need to do, because the work rarely stops on its own. We must be intentional about hitting the pause button so we can experience renewal, avoid burnout, and show up as the best version of ourselves. One study showed that, in the United States, more than half of workers didn't use their allotted vacation time. About a third of workers reported that they don't take time off to demonstrate their dedication to their jobs. But this pace is not sustainable. According to a professor in clinical psychology, overwork has become a "public health issue" in the United States.[13] So don't hesitate to use those vacation days, and take a mental health day when you need it.

Modeling Rest

I'm intentional about modeling healthy habits to my kids in terms of exercise and fueling my body with nourishing foods. I'm intentional about the way I speak about my body and how I respond when I look in the mirror, because I want to model positive self-image for them. I'm intentional about not talking about my weight or what foods I "should" or "shouldn't" be eating. I'm intentional about sharing how I manage my stress and emotions through deep breathing, prayer, gratitude, Pilates, journaling, and getting outside. I also want to be intentional about how I model rest.

The truth is, the people around us are watching the way we balance our days. Honoring our need for rest will have a positive impact not only on our individual health but also on those around us. When we take time for rest, we show others that it's okay for them to rest too. We show them that there's more to life than productivity. We show them that our bodies have limits and it's our job to honor and listen to those needs. When we do, we show others that we're worth taking care of—and so are they.

Rest is an aspect of wellness that's often overlooked. While most programs push you to do more, more, more, I'm here to remind you that you are a human being, with needs that are worth honoring—year to year, month to month, and day to day.

Put It into Practice

- **Start your morning** with five to ten minutes of prayer, meditation, Scripture reading, or deep breathing to begin the day with a calm, rested mind. (See the end of the chapter for a guided breathing exercise.)

- **Listen to your body's cues** throughout the day. When you feel tired, take a few minutes to sit in silence or lie down instead of pushing through.

- **Carve out thirty to sixty minutes** in your week to truly rest your body and mind by taking a nap, reading a feel-good book, or relaxing with a cup of tea and a beautiful view.

- **Set a timer** for one hour before bed to remind you to turn off screens and prepare your body for a good night of sleep.

- **The next time you dedicate space for rest,** tell your family or a friend so they'll be reminded that they are human and worthy of rest too.

Guided relaxation exercise

 Need a little help slowing down? Pop in your earbuds, scan the QR code, and listen to this guided relaxation. I'll lead you through a period of breathing exercises to help you quiet your mind and calm your body. Find a comfortable space to relax, and let's get started.

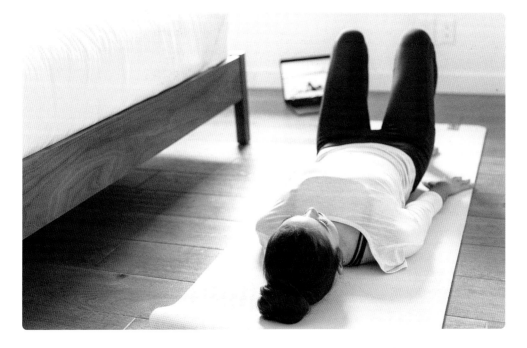

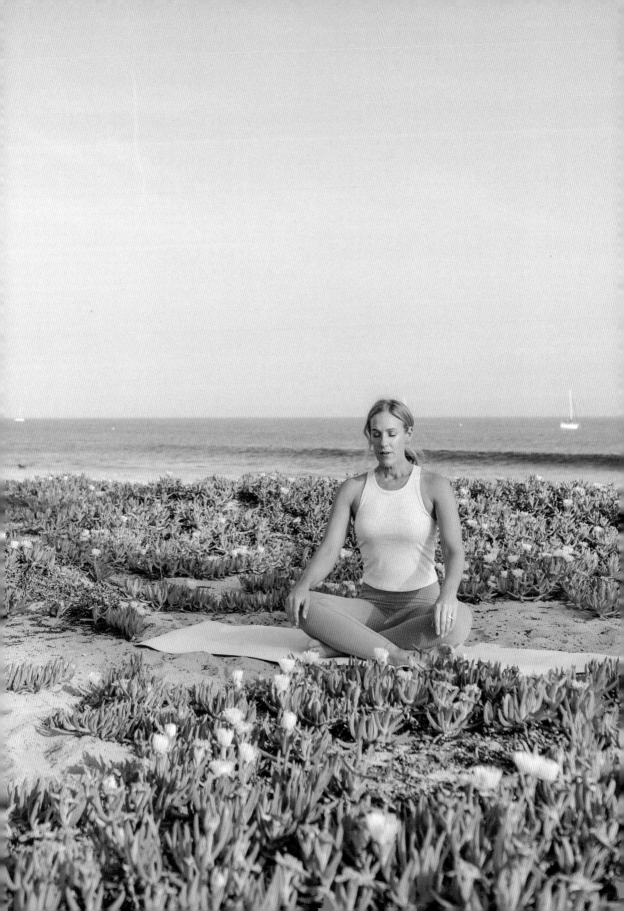

breathe

> Breathing is the
> first act of life,
> and the last.
> Our very life
> depends on it.
>
> Joseph Pilates

My journey with anxiety began in my early twenties. While I once had a carefree spirit, I became nervous, scared, and anxious as I entered the world of adulthood. Despite the many blessings in my life, I felt fearful and overwhelmed every day. I couldn't sleep, I struggled to stay present in the moment, and I was constantly worried.

When I was working in my first job, I started experiencing some mysterious health symptoms. I had unexplained aches and pains, and I went to doctor after doctor looking for answers. My tests continually came back "normal." I remember sitting in yet another doctor's office sharing my concerns (some about the physical symptoms themselves and some stemming from the fear that something was seriously wrong and it wasn't being diagnosed).

After a few minutes of half-hearted listening, the doctor crossed his arms and leaned against the counter. "Robin, you're what we call an enigma," he said. He then walked toward the door and told me to call again if my symptoms got worse.

This dismissal only heightened my fears. Not only was I worried about what was going on in my body, I now felt like I had nowhere to turn. If medical experts couldn't help me, what was I supposed to do?

My anxiety continued to spiral. I regularly woke up in a panic in the middle of the night, fearful that I wouldn't live to see the next day. I googled my symptoms to try to find answers, which only left me more terrified.

It was a vicious cycle, and my worries began to interfere with my day-to-day life. I couldn't concentrate on my work; I was nervous about ordinary activities. I could barely remember what it was like to live without being paralyzed by fear. I didn't feel like myself, and I wondered if my life would ever be the same again.

It was during this season that I took my first Pilates class. At the time, I had only a vague awareness of Pilates. I'd heard it was good for back pain (one of the many symptoms I was experiencing), so I figured I'd give it a try. I booked a class at a local studio, hoping it would help ease my pain. I had no idea it would provide so much more than that.

During that first class, in a studio above a downtown Starbucks, I remember lying on my back on a foam roller, gazing into the rafters. The instructor told us to take a big inhale. Then, on the exhale, we were to melt our shoulders over the foam roller and toward the ground. In that moment, I discovered just how much stress I'd been holding in my body. In one simple movement, my tension began to dissolve. It was like using a valve to release pressure I didn't know I had.

I ended the class feeling calmer, less stressed, and more in control. Of course, my clinical anxiety didn't disappear overnight, but as I walked out of the studio, I felt like I'd just discovered a tool that could dramatically change my life.

I was right.

Breath and Pilates

It took me a while to understand what makes the Pilates method uniquely powerful and transformative. I had exercised for years, but there was something different about the way I felt when I finished a Pilates workout. I'd go into class feeling tired, anxious, and unmotivated, and I'd walk out feeling the exact opposite.

I've come to understand that the combination of exercises, which restore balance, strength, and alignment, along with the intentional focus on breath, reaps benefits far beyond other forms of exercise.

Life depends on our ability to breathe, but the quality of life depends on our ability to breathe well.

During Pilates workouts, we use breath to connect our minds to our bodies and to get the most out of each exercise. Breathing deeply and effectively during Pilates workouts allows more oxygen to reach the muscles and the brain, which improves the way we feel and function. Joseph Pilates referred to this as an "internal shower"[1]—a way to flush out debris and toxins that accumulate in our bodies.

When you use breath to facilitate movement and connect your mind to your muscles, it not only improves the effectiveness of your workout but also leaves you feeling invigorated after you leave the mat. I have come to appreciate breath as a tool not only in Pilates but also in my everyday life.

Breath and the Body

Have you ever considered how many miraculous things take place in our bodies on a moment-to-moment basis? The heart pumps just the right amount of blood needed for survival, the nerves send messages back and forth to the brain, and the digestive system breaks down food to support the functions of the body. These processes are happening right now, while we're not even conscious of it!

Every day, every hour, and every minute, your lungs inhale fresh oxygen and exhale carbon dioxide to keep you alive. That oxygen is used to support every fiber of your being. In James Nestor's book *Breath*, he digs into the history and research of breath. After conversations with a wide variety of doctors, scientists, and practitioners, he concludes, "No matter what we eat, how much we exercise, how resilient our genes are, how skinny or young or wise we are—none of it will matter unless we're breathing correctly. That's what these researchers discovered. The missing

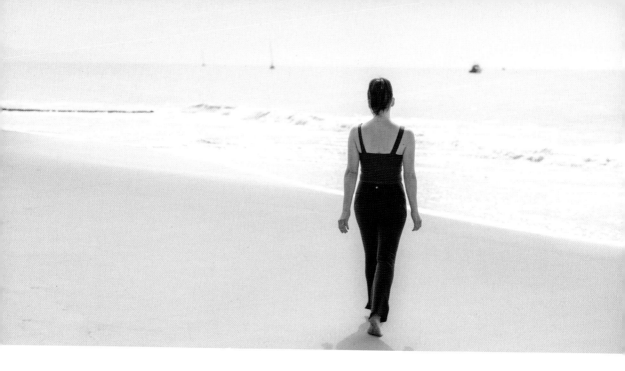

pillar in health is breath. It all starts there."[2] Put another way: life depends on our ability to breathe, but the quality of life depends on our ability to breathe well.

Breath isn't something that's discussed much in traditional health and fitness programs. But breathing properly may be one of the most powerful (and underutilized) tools in our wellness tool kit. Improving the way you breathe can have a significant impact on how you feel, as well as on measurable biomarkers of good health, such as hormonal balance, stress level, blood pressure, and heart rate variability.[3] On top of that, healthy breathing has been shown to decrease depression, anxiety, and stress, and it helps provide your body with the energy it needs to complete its functions.[4]

We may not have to stop and remember to breathe to stay alive (thank goodness!). But there are factors we control that impact the quality of our breath.

Poor posture compresses the diaphragm and restricts the lungs.

If you sit at a desk all day, look down at your devices, or have poor posture, your breathing is negatively impacted. Poor posture has an immediate effect on respiratory function, as it compromises the strength and effectiveness of the diaphragm (a dome-shaped muscle just below the lungs that's the primary muscle used in respiration).[5] Likewise, if you have scoliosis (like I do), your breathing can be impacted. Curves in the spine, whether because of posture or spinal position, restrict the movement of the lungs and diaphragm, which leads to shallow or incomplete breath cycles.

At the risk of sounding like a broken record, this is another reason Pilates can be a beneficial part of every person's wellness routine. Pilates promotes good posture by building core strength, lengthening the spine, and restoring balance to the body in terms of both alignment and musculature. Pilates helps you to become more aware of your posture throughout the day, which not only reduces aches, pains, and risk of injury, but also improves the quality of your breath.

A hurried mind leads to shallow and incomplete breaths.

When we hold our breath or take in short, shallow breaths, our bodies don't receive the oxygen required to function at optimal levels. Shallow breathing leaves us feeling tired, sluggish, and anxious. Studies show that our breathing can significantly affect the way we feel emotionally too. Unlike changing our diet, which may not produce tangible results for months, improving the way we breathe can bring a noticeable difference in minutes. When we learn to breathe effectively, we reap the benefits of relieved muscle tension, reduced stress, improved sleep, increased focus, and higher energy levels.

Shallow breathing happens for a variety of reasons. It may be due to poor posture or a hurried lifestyle. As we rush from task to task, check the latest notifications on our phones, and scroll through trending headlines, our breathing patterns tend to change. The next time you read something that makes you feel uneasy, take note of these patterns. You may catch yourself holding your breath or taking quick, shallow breaths.

Shallow breathing brings oxygen into the chest and the upper part of the lungs but doesn't allow the oxygen to fully reach the diaphragm or fill up the lungs. This can become a troubling cycle, as rapid, shallow breathing can be triggered by stressful situations and in turn induce a stress response in the nervous system. This sends the body into fight-or-flight mode, leaving us feeling even more stressed and anxious.

When I started making a conscious effort to connect with my body, I discovered that I hold my breath when I scroll Instagram. I found this curious and started digging further into this pattern. To my surprise, I found out that I'm not the only one who does this. Researcher Linda Stone identified a phenomenon called "email apnea." According to her study of more than two hundred participants, roughly 80

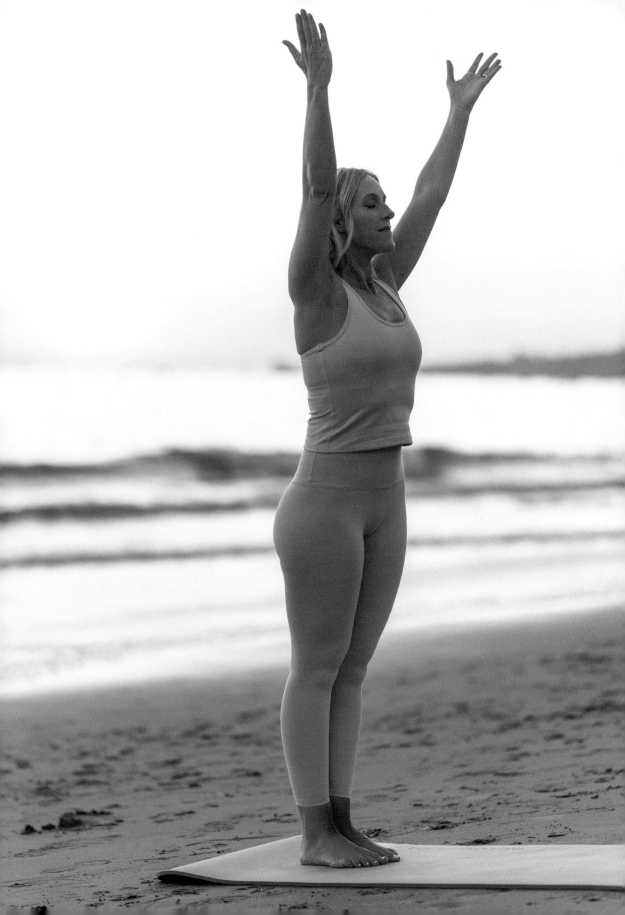

percent of people held their breath while reading email or scrolling their phones.[6] While this habit may seem harmless, it can have serious health ramifications in the long term, such as increased cortisol levels, lack of focus, and elevated heart rate.[7]

Mouth breathing is less effective than nasal breathing.

We all know a snorer. It's either someone you love . . . or you. Snoring is typically thought of as harmless, but it may be more significant than we think. Snoring is often a sign of mouth breathing, which occurs when air pathways are inflamed or misaligned. Inhaling and exhaling primarily through the mouth has been shown to have a negative effect on energy, dental health, cognition, and sleep.[8] When we inhale through the nose, in contrast, our bodies receive a boost of nitric oxide, which means we can absorb about 20 percent more oxygen than by breathing through the mouth alone. Nasal breathing also helps to purify the air we breathe, boosting our immune health.[9]

Learning how to breathe more effectively is a simple, free way to make significant improvements to your health and well-being. Start by becoming more aware of your breath and your breathing patterns throughout the day. Notice when you're holding your breath, breathing shallowly, or breathing through your mouth. You may also want to pursue exercise such as Pilates that focuses on the quality of your breathing. As you retrain your breathing during the day, you'll likely begin to see improvement while you're sleeping too. If you're concerned about your breathing or snoring and you aren't noticing any improvement, be sure to reach out to your health care provider.

Breath and the Nervous System

The way we breathe has a direct impact on the functions of the brain. The autonomic nervous system is responsible for regulating several functions in the body, including blood pressure, digestion, and respiratory rate. When we feel nervous, tense, scared, or panicked, our sympathetic nervous system takes over and our breath quickens. This is often called fight-or-flight mode. When we feel calm, relaxed, safe, and at ease, our parasympathetic nervous system is in control. In this state, our breath slows down, which allows us to take longer, deeper breaths. We can use deep breathing as a tool to calm our bodies and our minds, sending a signal of relaxation to our brains.

When my anxiety peaked in my early twenties, I became an extremely nervous flier. As soon as the plane took off, my palms started sweating, my heart began racing, and I felt like everything around me was spinning. Every time I flew, I was on the verge of a panic attack by the time the plane took off. Although I felt like I had no control over my spiraling thoughts, I realized there was one thing I could control: my breath. If I focused on my breath, I could change what was happening in my brain and help ward off panic. To this day, when the plane is taking off, you'll find me in my seat with my eyes closed and my noise-canceling headphones on, counting my breaths.

Breathing exercises are shown to stimulate the vagus nerve, a primary component of the parasympathetic nervous system (the part that calms us down). The vagus nerve is responsible for regulating functions such as heart rate, digestion, and respiratory rate. Studies have shown that stimulating the vagus nerve can support the treatment of depression, PTSD, and inflammatory bowel disease, as well as mood and anxiety disorders. It's also helpful in improving immune function and reducing inflammation.[10]

While movement, intentional breathing, and other lifestyle changes can significantly improve our physical and mental health, there are times when it's important to seek professional help. I've gone to counseling on and off for the past fifteen years, and I highly recommend therapy or counseling as part of any wellness routine. There's no shame in seeking help, and this is a vital part of experiencing whole-person health.

Breath Connects Us to Our Bodies

As you become aware of your breathing, it will become easier to listen to your body's cues and respond accordingly. Utilizing our breath for better health is free and accessible—it requires nothing more than awareness and intentionality.

As you go through your day, be aware of your breathing. When you feel stressed, angry, or overwhelmed, calm your nervous system by taking five to ten slow, deep breaths. (I've been known to declare a "mommy breathing break" when I'm on the brink of losing it. I make a loud announcement to all who can hear and lock myself in my room for a few minutes to focus on my breath to calm myself down.)

During your Pilates workout (or your workout of choice), pay attention as you inhale and exhale. If you notice that your breath is becoming shallow, take it as a cue to slow down, adjust your posture, and breathe deeply again.

If you feel disconnected from your body after illness, injury, or trauma, or if you're feeling tired and depleted, set aside a few minutes a day to close your eyes and focus on your breath. When I teach Pilates workouts, I encourage my class to use their breath when it gets hard. We can do the same in our daily lives.

When you're mindful about proper breathing, and when you take opportunities to focus on breathwork throughout the day, you'll start to feel the positive effects on your mind and body—often within a matter of minutes.[11] You will find yourself gaining equilibrium, starting at the center of your being and flowing into every area of your life.

Put It into Practice

- **Set reminders** for yourself throughout the day to focus on good posture, which supports optimal breathing. You might want to set your phone alarm to go off at a time when you're usually feeling tired. This is a good nudge to realign yourself and take a few deep breaths.

- **Incorporate Pilates** into your weekly routine to improve your posture and restore optimal alignment.

- **Create a mental trigger** to remind you to pause and notice your breathing. This could be when you're sitting at a red light, anytime your phone rings, or just before you eat a meal (bonus: this helps with mindfulness, too!).

- **Breathe through your nose** as often as possible (and especially at night!). If you're concerned about snoring or sleep apnea, reach out to your doctor to schedule a sleep study.

- **Next time you're feeling anxious, angry, or nervous**, take five to ten deep belly breaths to change your physiological state and restore your nervous system to a place of calm.

Breathing Techniques

If you want to incorporate a few breathing exercises into your daily routine, here are a few you can implement right away.

Simple Breathing Exercise

This is a simple exercise I use when I'm feeling nervous or stressed during the day, or when I'm simply looking for a way to calm my mind and relax.

1. Inhale through the nose for a count of six.

2. Exhale through the mouth for a count of eight.

3. If you're feeling panicked or short of breath, start with a count of four and work your way up.

Bubble-Blowing Breathing Exercise

This exercise works well for adults and children. I walk my daughter through this exercise when she's feeling worried or anxious, and it helps her calm her nervous system and quiet her mind.

1. Inhale through the nose for a count of five.

2. When you exhale, imagine that you're blowing bubbles through a straw.

3. Each time you exhale, imagine a colored bubble floating away and then popping. (For example, you might picture sparkly pink bubbles, bright-red bubbles, or black-and-white polka-dot bubbles.)

Square Breathing Exercise

This exercise includes a tactical component to help you connect your mind and your body. This is beneficial to do when you're stressed during a meeting, when you're nervous while taking a test, or any time panicky feelings arise.

1. As you breathe, draw a square with a finger on your thigh.

2. Inhale through the nose to a count of five as you draw one side of the square, hold for five as you draw the next side, exhale for five as you draw the third side, and rest for five.

3. Continue until you feel calm and recentered.

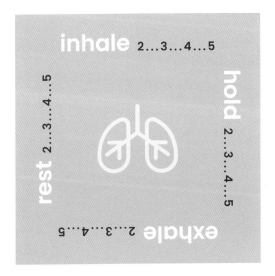

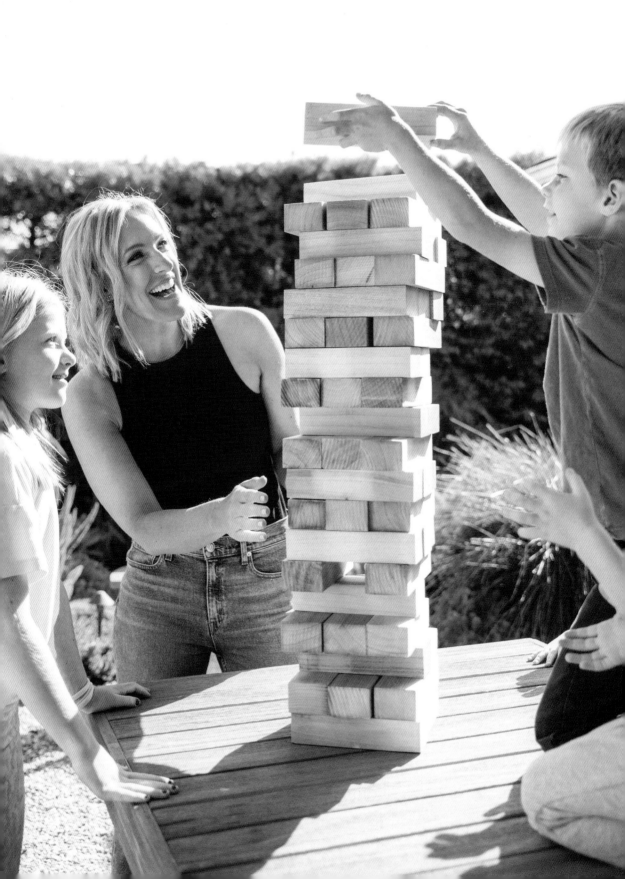

play

We don't stop playing
because we grow old;
we grow old because
we stop playing.

George Bernard Shaw

After a particularly challenging few years of adjusting to life with twins, navigating a worldwide pandemic, working from home, and doing school at home, Matt and I realized that fun had left the building. We'd become so focused on what needed to happen to get through the day that doing anything outside the daily routine was moved to the back burner. Like much of the world, we were in survival mode. The days began to blur together. The snack requests were constant, and the lineup of dishes that needed to be washed was never ending.

On an uneventful, foggy day, as I was washing dishes and wiping down

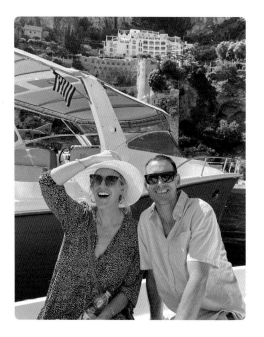

counters, I looked at Matt across the room and realized it had been months since I'd heard his laugh. I tried to conjure up the memory in my head—the sound of his true, contagious belly laughter—and realized I had to dig far back to access it.

As I continued to scrub the spilled smoothie from the counter, I realized I wasn't sure when I'd last laughed either. Our moods were flat; our zest for life was low. We needed more levity—as individuals and as a family.

Around the same time, I received the order from my doctor to lower my stress level. It was clear that something needed to change.

I scheduled a babysitter and took Matt on a date to a coffee shop down the street. We had exactly one hour together before we had to return home, and I was determined to use this time to tackle our challenge head on. I channeled my initial sadness and disappointment into fuel for making a change.

In our joggers and sweatshirts, over steamy Americanos, I shared how I was feeling. I told him that I missed his smile and the sound of his laughter—and my own, too. While this was hard for him to hear, he didn't disagree. The demands of daily life were weighing on us, and we were both in a funk.

As we sipped our coffee in the late-morning sunshine, we talked about how we could have more fun—not the manufactured version of fun, but the kind of fun that makes you laugh until your belly hurts, scream with excitement, and remember what it feels like to be truly alive. That day we committed to making a change.

As with most worthwhile endeavors, change didn't happen overnight. It was a challenging process to figure out how to interrupt our daily routine to pursue more fun during a demanding season, when free time was limited and stress levels were high. But we were determined.

We brainstormed activities we really enjoyed and carved out time in our monthly schedule to do more of those things. We included space in our budget for expenses that weren't necessarily practical, and we asked for help with our kids so we could go away together. I pushed through my fear of trying new things so I could remember what it felt like to live life to the fullest.

Intentionally pursuing play led us to take a ski trip (returning to the slopes after fifteen years!), ride snowmobiles, take salsa dancing lessons, ride Jet Skis, go four-wheeling, ride electric bikes along the beach, challenge one another to intense games of four square in our cul-de-sac, swing from a giant trapeze on a pier near our home, and take an acro-yoga class that made us laugh until we cried. Many days, choosing play was as simple as saying yes to a board game with our kids or jumping in the pool instead of sitting on the sidelines.

Health isn't always about pushing harder, drumming up more willpower, or following strict rules. Isn't that a relief? We aren't just bodies to fix; we are souls to be nurtured. Our physical, mental, and emotional well-being is impacted by how much we play—that is, how much we engage in activities simply for recreation and pleasure. While this may seem like an easy component of wellness to embrace, you may be neglecting this area more than you realize (like I was!).

> Loosening up and having fun can—
> and should—be an intentional part
> of your wellness routine.

As I've gotten older and my responsibilities have increased, I've taken on the approach of work first, play later. I figure if I get things done first, I can use whatever time is left for recreation and pleasure. But the reality is, the work is rarely finished. There's always something practical that needs to be attended to. When we wait to get it all done before we take time to play, at best we'll sneak a tiny bit of recreation into the crevices, and at worst the play will never happen.

A life without play is a life out of balance. Just as we take time to plan our workouts and fuel our bodies with nourishing foods, we also need to make space for play. Doing so is not frivolous; it's essential.

Loosening up and having fun can—and should—be an intentional part of your wellness routine. It's yet another tool to become the healthiest version of yourself and to truly live life to the fullest.

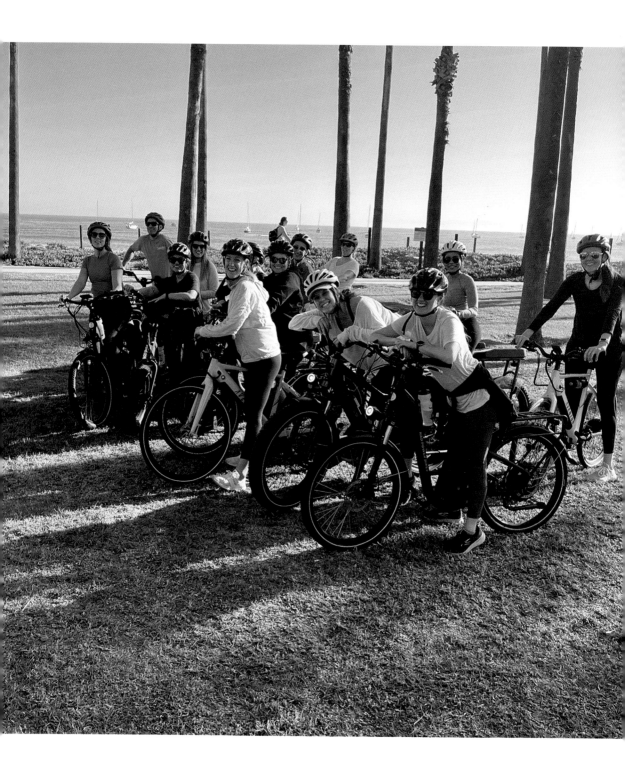

Making time for play can do the following:

- increase your happiness
- support heart health
- improve mental clarity
- boost energy
- improve focus
- strengthen relationships[1]

A key component of play is that we do it purely for the sake of enjoyment, not for an end result. Play can look different for everyone, so it's important to find your unique style. For some, it may be singing karaoke, while for others it may mean taking a painting class, playing cards, going for a bike ride, or playing pickleball.

Take a moment to reflect on what play looks like for you. Think about how you played in the past (as a child or a young adult). Then consider how you play today. If you're coming up blank, don't worry. By the end of this chapter, you'll feel inspired and equipped to pursue play with a renewed sense of purpose.

More Play, Less Stress

Before we made an intentional commitment to play more, Matt and I were not only feeling bored but also lacking connection in our relationship. We spent a lot of time together but had fallen into a rut. Making play a priority helped us rekindle our relationship and our appreciation for each other.

The reality is, life can be hard, and the days can feel long. When we engage in play, it provides an opportunity to step away from work, stress, and our daily responsibilities. It gives our minds a break and creates a chance to unplug, have fun, and let go. On a physiological level, play allows our bodies to release more endorphins (the feel-good hormones), and it lowers stress hormones.

Studies have shown that those who play more and take a more fun-filled approach to life find it easier to cope with stress.[2] According to Lynn Barnett, professor of recreation, sports, and tourism at the University of Illinois at Urbana-Champaign, "Highly playful adults feel the same stressors as anyone else, but they appear to experience and react to them differently, allowing stressors to roll off more easily than those who are less playful."[3] Our ability to manage stress is central to our well-being, especially as stress rates skyrocket in our world.

Play Improves Productivity

Ever wonder why the top tech companies fill their office space with Ping-Pong tables and host foosball tournaments on Fridays? They know that providing opportunities to play not only supports their employees' mental health and job satisfaction but also improves their quality of work. Play increases focus, productivity, creativity, and problem-solving skills.[4] Bringing a spirit of playfulness into your life is good for your health and the health of those around you—and it's also good for your career.

When my friend Karli worked in the biology lab at a local university, the professors (all well-respected, esteemed academics) had ongoing prank wars between classes, lectures, and research. When they weren't solving the world's big scientific problems, they were hiding under desks, decorating offices with tinfoil, and sneaking frogs into desk drawers. It's no surprise that their job satisfaction was high. But they were also making significant contributions in the world of science.

Play and work don't have to be (and shouldn't be!) mutually exclusive. Whether that means adding levity to long days of meetings, sharing funny texts and images, or playing friendly pranks on coworkers, keeping a playful spirit is good for health, productivity, work, and relationships—all at the same time!

The Best Anti-Aging Hack

It's a gift to grow old—each year we live on earth is an absolute privilege. Along with that comes a desire to age well. We want to maintain our vitality and stay strong in body and mind. One of the most underrated ways to stay young at heart and to slow the aging process is by having more fun and laughing more often.

Research has shown that laughter is medicine, for both the soul and the body. Health care professionals agree that laughter can reduce stress, ease pain, lift moods, improve the immune system, and send more oxygen to the organs of the body. Laughter lowers cortisol levels and increases endorphins, which is beneficial for mental health.[5]

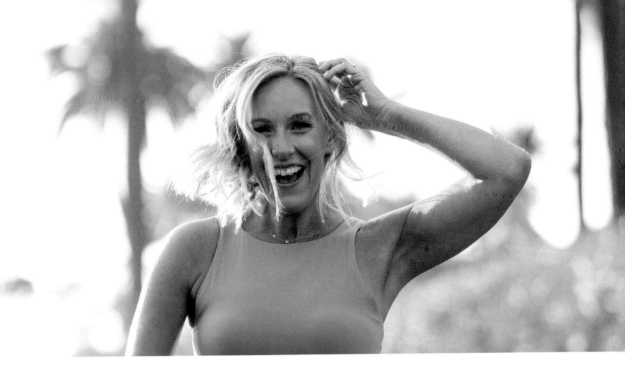

Like play, laughter improves brain connectivity and activates the pleasure center in the brain. It releases serotonin, which can reduce symptoms of depression.[6] It has even been shown to improve blood flow and reduce inflammation for those with inflammatory diseases such as rheumatoid arthritis.[7]

While laughter is not a cure-all, it has a positive impact on your well-being, regardless of the health challenges you face. It's free, accessible, enjoyable, and best of all, contagious in the best way! Finding ways to laugh may take some effort, but the investment is worthwhile—for your own wellness and for the people around you. (As long as they think you're funny too—something I'm still working on with my kids!)

Choosing a Playful Mindset

When you're an adult with a calendar full of chores and responsibilities, life has a way of getting monotonous. It's easy to fall into familiar patterns instead of embracing a playful approach to life. But play doesn't have to involve expensive hobbies or big trips; it can be about small choices and the way you view life.

Depending on the season you're in, choosing a playful mindset might look like going to the dog park with your dog instead of going for your usual, uneventful stroll. It might mean choosing shows and movies that lift your spirit and make you

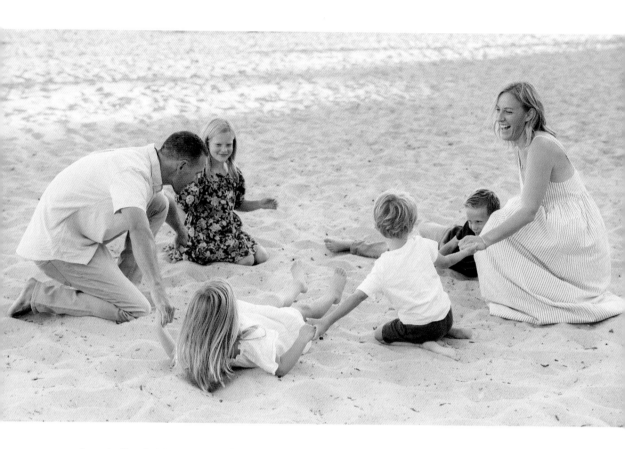

laugh. It might mean taking up a new hobby or joining a local kickball league to help you feel like a kid again (bonus: this will also help you unplug, connect with others, and move your body). When you're planning time away, you could take trips that include opportunities for play and adventure, such as kayaking, sledding, dancing, or even a trip to an amusement park.

Part of embracing a playful spirit means not taking yourself too seriously. It's okay (and helpful!) to laugh at yourself. When we laugh at ourselves, we lighten our load, lift our mood, and change our entire approach to life.

When I teach a particularly challenging exercise in Pilates class, or one that can feel awkward to execute, people may feel frustrated or discouraged at first. This can lead to a spiral of negative self-talk, all because of one silly Pilates exercise. But that thought spiral can be interrupted when we laugh at ourselves and remember that it's just Pilates. We gain perspective, which allows us to stay in a place of enjoyment and keep moving forward. This principle holds true in the rest of life too. The more we laugh at ourselves, the better we're able to handle the challenges that come our way.

Just as you fuel your body with nourishing food, you can fuel your perspective with play, laughter, and fun. Play is accessible to all, regardless of age, budget, or schedule. It isn't a luxury; it's an essential ingredient to living well.

Put It into Practice

- **Break out of your daily routine** by trying something new (such as stand-up paddleboarding, salsa lessons, rock skipping, or camping). Try not to take yourself too seriously in the process.

- **Volunteer to play** with animals at a local shelter.

- **Create an obstacle course** in your backyard, put together a puzzle, or turn on some music and dance.

- **Schedule a monthly game night** with family or friends. (Bonus points for games that make you laugh!)

- **Download or stream something funny.** Listening to a funny podcast or watching a stand-up comedy series can take your mind off a busy day and help you enjoy a good laugh.

- **Schedule a date** with your funniest friend.

- **Play a good-natured prank** on someone. Consider hiding behind the corner and scaring your friend or placing a rubber bug on your spouse's side of the bed. This type of play brings you back to childhood and can fill your home or workplace with more levity (when done thoughtfully, of course). Good-natured pranks add laughter into your life and improve your mood in a matter of minutes.

Jackie H.

For the past several years I've made my home in Richmond, Virginia, with my two lovable pups, Garbanzo and Max. Play hasn't always been a priority for me—in fact, it was quite the opposite when I was growing up. I was encouraged to pursue academics and certain extracurriculars, and it was typical for me to do homework on Friday night, perform at violin recitals on the weekend, and participate in golf tournaments and tutoring during the summer.

As an adult, I found that my hobbies felt more like work—something else I had to get done. And because many of my hobbies involved performing, I was easily discouraged by others' negative input. Basically, all the joy was taken out of what was supposed to be fun.

I've come to realize that my whole well-being is a priority and that part of becoming my healthiest self includes making time for fun and laughter—things that don't feel like work. So now I pursue play simply for the joy of it! I joined a kickball team, and I went on a solo snowboarding trip. I take improv classes, stand-up comedy classes, and online singing lessons. And anytime I take my dogs to the park, I'm guaranteed to have a good time. Watching them play gets

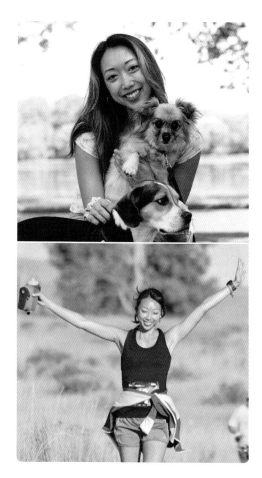

me in a playful mood and inspires me to have fun myself.

Embracing play and laughter has helped me meet new people, develop friendships, and discover what I truly enjoy (and what I don't!). It gives me things to look forward to and helps me find more balance and joy. I'm learning to believe that my needs truly matter—and that we all need to have fun! Prioritizing play is one more piece of the puzzle in becoming my healthiest self.

Chapter 10

choose

Every moment
of our life can be
the beginning
of great things.

Joseph Pilates

Did you know that you make somewhere in the ballpark of 35,000 decisions in a single day?[1] I don't know about you, but just seeing that number makes me exhausted. While it can seem taxing to face so many decisions each day, this also presents an opportunity.

You might feel like your life is stuck in a rut or like someone else—a boss or a parent or a spouse—calls some shots in your life. But the truth is, every one of us has a superpower of sorts: the ability to choose. When it comes to our health, true transformation happens when we recognize and embrace this gift.

By this point in the book, my hope is

that you have a deeper understanding of what it means to pursue true wellness. Being well and living life to the fullest goes far beyond the size of our jeans, the shape of our thighs, or the number on the scale. True wellness includes both the body and the mind, affecting everything from our ability to move through life with energy and strength to our emotional well-being and our overall life satisfaction.

The way we feel impacts our relationships, our creativity, and our ability to pursue goals and engage in the activities we enjoy. When we break free from outdated, restrictive habits from the past and embrace a holistic approach to wellness, we're able to remain grounded, connect our bodies and our minds, discover our true strength, breathe more deeply, and stand up taller.

I've experienced this transformation in my own life. Before I embraced this approach, I lived in a constant state of striving—feeling guilty about the workouts I wasn't doing or the food I should or shouldn't be eating. I was fixated on metrics, and my headspace was filled with negative thoughts about my body. The simple act of getting dressed often resulted in feelings of disgust, frustration, and insecurity. While I still have days when I feel bloated or uncomfortable in my body, like every woman does, I now have a clearer picture of my worth and what it means to be well—and I have tools to reframe my thoughts before I fall into a shame spiral.

Freeing up this headspace allows me to invest more time, energy, and attention in what matters most to me—my children, my husband, my dreams, and my goal to make a positive impact on the world around me. Now I live in freedom from guilt, shame, and the exhausting expectation to look a certain way. The negative thoughts still creep in now and then. But at my core, I have a much deeper and more meaningful understanding of what it means to be truly well—to be well to the core. This is a gift I hope you will embrace too.

Rewiring Your Brain

Embracing this new approach is not a quick fix; it's a lifelong endeavor. Changing the way you think requires intentionality and daily decisions. But over time, these choices will rewire your brain, replacing your old default settings with new, healthy patterns.

The brain's ability to change and adapt is called neuroplasticity. When thoughts cycle in our heads over and over or when we repeat certain patterns, neural pathways are created in the brain. The more these thoughts or habits are repeated, the stronger the neural pathways become, until this is our default way of thinking or behaving. If you keep wanting to change but feel stuck, this is why. The good news is that through neuroplasticity, we can create new neural pathways and change the way our brains function.[2] The more we choose healthy ways of thinking, the easier it becomes.[3]

Now that your eyes are opened to this new way of caring for yourself, you'll notice habits and thought patterns that don't fit with this new approach. For example, you may catch yourself equating the size and shape of your body with the state of your health. You may recognize when you're falling into an all or nothing mentality with your workouts. You may notice when you're focusing on what you want to "fix" about your appearance instead of how you want to feel.

> The more we choose healthy ways of thinking,
> the easier it becomes.

Just recently I was preparing for a photo shoot, and I felt my old way of thinking creep in. As I tried on outfits, I started thinking, *My thighs look so big. Ugh, you can see my cellulite in these pants. My body doesn't look as thin as it used to—people are going to notice that I've gained weight.*

If I'm not intentional, I put pressure on myself to look a certain way, especially because fitness instructors are supposed to look a certain way. Thankfully, I've learned to become more conscious of these destructive thought patterns over time.

As I looked in the mirror, I was able to out these statements as untrue (or simply irrelevant) and replace them with what I know to be true—and more important, thoughts that align with the person I want to be and the impact I want to have.

In every season, I want to show up as the woman I am, embracing the body I have and pursuing a balanced approach to health, fitness, and wellness. And I want to support other women so they can do the same.

I reminded myself that my worth is not found in the size and shape of my body, and that I'm worthy and accepted, just as I am.

When you notice old thought patterns that no longer serve you, don't beat yourself up. Simply recognize them without judgment. Then be intentional about reframing them and choosing a better way.

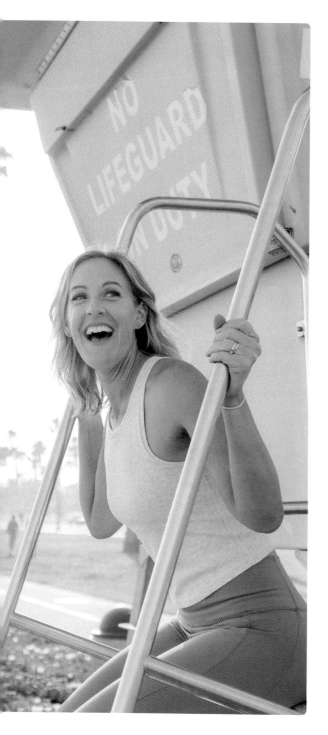

One way to change your default patterns is to journal about what you're telling yourself and compare that to what you actually believe—or want to believe. For example, before my photo shoot, the story I started telling myself was that I needed to lose weight and look thinner before I got in front of the camera. But when I called that story out and reflected on it, it didn't hold up. What I value isn't wearing a certain clothing size or obtaining a culturally approved body type. I want to live out (and teach) an approach that incorporates mental and physical health—*true* health, which also means freedom from shame and self-loathing. When I wrote down my thoughts, it was easier to spot the lies in my thinking, reframe the situation, and clarify my priorities.

Choose the Kind of Person You Want to Be

How can we change the world for women and girls so we as a society can restore our relationship with exercise, food, and our bodies? This may sound like a daunting prospect, but big transformation starts small and close to home. When we change our thoughts, we change our behaviors—and as a result, we change the world. It starts with us.

From this day forward, you have

a choice. You can continue to operate out of your default habits, patterns, and behaviors, or you can become the type of person you want to be. Creating a vision for your life is an important step in ensuring that you don't just read the words on these pages but live them out. Transformation occurs when you shift your focus from where you are now to the woman you want to be and then make decisions that align with that vision.

Take a moment to consider what you believe about yourself and how those beliefs align with your self-talk and daily habits. For example, maybe you've always believed that you're the type of person who just doesn't like to exercise. Or maybe you see yourself as someone who doesn't have a lot of willpower or doesn't like to eat healthy foods. Pause and ask yourself, *What beliefs do I currently have about myself that are holding me back from being the type of person I want to be?*

Chances are, it's time for an identity tune-up. What we believe about ourselves is who we eventually become.

Choose to Invest in Your Health

After working with women for more than a decade, I continue to be struck by how hesitant we are to invest in ourselves. We drop plenty of money on our kids and our pets, but we often deliberate for days about spending money on things that are beneficial for us. We spend our time helping other people, working long hours, and volunteering, but we hesitate to take a few hours just for ourselves. I see this in women I teach, and I see it in myself, too.

As women, we're conditioned from a young age to put others' needs before our own. And while I'm a big believer in serving others, I've learned that we can't love people well when we're running on empty ourselves. When we don't feel good, it's hard to take action on others' behalf. When we're exhausted, it's hard to remain patient and kind. When we haven't created space and time to fulfill our own basic needs (such as movement, sleep, and nourishment), it's harder to make a positive impact on the people we love.

Here's the hard lesson I've learned over the years: no one can do this for you. Rarely will your boss step in on your behalf to make sure you're taking time off for your mental health. It's highly unlikely that someone will be watching the clock to ensure that you're getting enough sleep, and no one can do the workout for you. No one will remind you to breathe well or incorporate play into your routine or find ways to recharge your emotional batteries. It's up to you to ensure that you are prioritizing your own wellness.

You are worth investing in. You are worthy, just as you are right now. You are beautifully and wonderfully made, and it's not a luxury to care for your mind and body; it's a necessity. Investing in your health and well-being doesn't have to look like a day at the spa (as lovely as that might be). It's about making decisions that contribute to your wellness, starting today. These can be small investments, such as drinking more water throughout the day, or significant investments, such as working through long-held false beliefs in therapy.

Investing in ourselves when we are pulled in many other directions isn't always easy, but it's always worth it. *You* are worth it.

Choose to Create New Habits

Whether we realize it or not, we repeat behaviors—day after day and week after week. The brain utilizes more energy than any other organ in the body.[4] In an effort to conserve energy and perform all its necessary functions, it relies on certain habits or behaviors that can be done without thinking. For example, we don't have to consciously process the way we brush our teeth each day. We don't have to actively think through the steps of washing dishes—we've done it enough times that neural pathways in our brains make it easy and efficient to repeat these behaviors.

This is how habits develop. Some are intentional, and others are not. Some we're aware of, and others have become such a part of who we are and what we do that we don't even notice them. Once you're clear about your values and goals, you can start creating new habits to help you become the person you want to be.

Here are a few tips to help you experience success in forming healthy habits:

Start small. If you've always assumed that workouts need to be long, you may scoff at the recommendation to embrace ten-minute workouts. But it's common to start off too ambitious and then lose traction before you've had time to truly build the new habit. When you start small, it's easier to say yes when life gets busy, which allows you to feel successful. That feeling of success trains the brain to repeat the behavior, leading to a new habit that can be built on in the future.

Celebrate. When we celebrate progress and acknowledge our efforts and accomplishments no matter how small, hormones are released that help encode the new behavior into our brains, making us more likely to repeat it.[5] That's why every Pilates workout I teach includes an intentional pause to celebrate that you took time out of your day to care for your health. It's also why the Lindywell app includes fun features to help you celebrate each time you work out. Not only does celebration make for a more enjoyable experience, it's proven to help build the habit of consistency as you work toward your goals.

Find support and accountability. Research shows that people who have accountability are far more likely to stick with a habit than those who don't.[6] When you surround yourself with support, you receive cues that trigger the new behavior you're trying to make into a habit. Maybe you have a friend who invites you to go on a walk with her, or maybe you swap healthy dinner recipes with a friend, or maybe you get encouragement from someone in your community with similar values and goals. This journey isn't meant to be walked alone; we all need people who will kindly nudge us toward the habits we're trying to build so we can become the healthiest version of ourselves.

Choose to Be an Example of True Health

As I've shared this message of whole-person wellness for the past decade, it has felt like swimming upstream at times. This is a countercultural approach—it's not the language most people speak when they talk about health and fitness. I know that if I'd posted more "before and after" photos on my Instagram account, made more weight-loss claims on my website, photoshopped pictures of myself, or wore myself out trying to get my body into an "ideal" shape, I'd likely have sold more subscriptions or received more attention. But I have a personal responsibility and a deep conviction to tell the truth and pave a new path for women around the world—a path that leads to true wellness rather than constant striving.

This challenge isn't a theoretical one for me. As I've navigated this tension in my work, I've also been navigating it in my own life, in friendships, and in social settings.

As your eyes are opened to this new approach to health, fitness, and wellness, you'll notice how many conversations around weight, bodies, food, and diet center on faulty assumptions. These conversations are often a way to bond and connect with other women, and when you don't lean in because you're working to choose a different path, it may feel awkward at times.

But in these moments, you have an opportunity to set an example of grace over guilt and exhibit the freedom you've found. Sometimes this might look like sharing directly with your friends and addressing the conversation head-on, and other times a smile and a gentle change of subject may be the best approach. Either way, people will notice a difference in your outlook—and be inspired.

I also want to be intentional about the example I'm setting for the next generation. I don't want my children to hear me complain about my body or talk about how I shouldn't eat certain foods. Even when they don't seem to be paying attention, they are always listening and watching. I'm careful about the media they consume too —I'm mindful of avoiding shows or advertisements that promote an unhealthy view of the body.

As a Pilates instructor, I am intentional about the words I use and the messages I convey while I'm teaching. I know that my words are heard not just by the person doing the workout but also by other ears in the room. This is a privilege and responsibility that I don't take lightly. Whether you realize it or not, the children and teens in your life are learning how to navigate the world by watching what you say and do. What an opportunity we have to change the world the next generation grows up in. We can be part of creating an environment where our children, grandchildren, nieces, nephews, and friends can honor and respect their bodies, being grateful for what their bodies can do.

Can you imagine if we all made a conscious choice to stop the negative talk about our bodies or the foods we should or shouldn't eat? Think about how much headspace would be freed up if we stopped worrying about the ways our bodies don't measure up or how we should push harder, do more, or be more like someone else. What if instead we accepted and respected the bodies we have today? We'd be able to let go of judgment and lift one another up, freeing ourselves to spend our time and energy on what truly matters.

We have a choice. We have an opportunity to live out a holistic, realistic, balanced approach to health and wellness in our homes, workplaces, and communities. We have the power to change the conversation—and when we change the

Choose grace over guilt

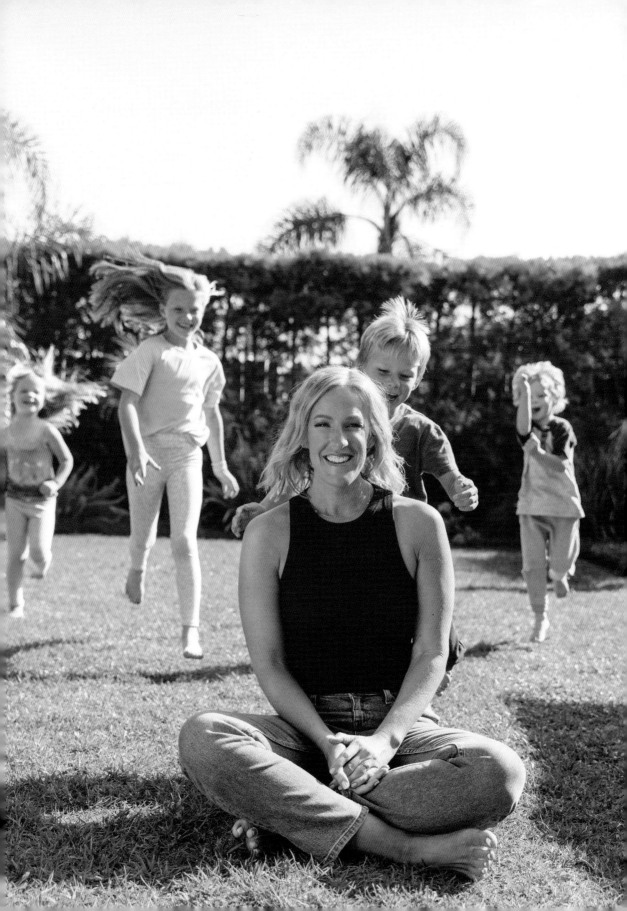

conversation, we can change the world. As we focus on progress over perfection, choose grace over guilt, connect with our bodies, and respond to our needs, we inspire those around us to do the same. When other people see us celebrate progress (no matter how small) and honor the season we're in, they will believe they can do the same.

Choose to Be Kind to Yourself

As you move forward with a refreshed vision of the person you want to become and renewed motivation to become well to the core, remember to be kind to yourself. Perfection isn't required to make progress. You will undoubtedly have days when you feel inspired, motivated, and aligned, and there will be other days when you feel challenged, discouraged, and exhausted. There will be times you fall into old habits and patterns and need to refocus and reset. That's okay—it's all part of the journey toward lifelong wellness.

You now have ten components of mind-body wellness to incorporate into your daily routines to help you to pursue health in a way that takes your whole self into account and helps you show up as the healthiest, most vibrant version of yourself and live life to the fullest.

Here are the ten components:

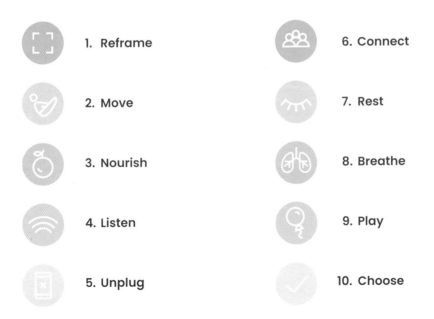

1. Reframe

2. Move

3. Nourish

4. Listen

5. Unplug

6. Connect

7. Rest

8. Breathe

9. Play

10. Choose

These components work together to create momentum and synergy, propelling you forward on your journey to be well to the core. Remember—it's all about small changes. As these decisions add up, you will find freedom to embrace the season you're in and the seasons that lie ahead.

As you navigate the ebbs and flows of this new approach, remember that every day provides an opportunity to start fresh. Every hour provides an opportunity to recenter. Every moment provides an opportunity to choose a new thought that supports your vision for who you want to become. So take a deep breath, stand tall, relax your shoulders, and remember: you're worth it.

✓ Put It into Practice

- **Start your day** by visualizing the person you want to become. As the day progresses, aim to make decisions that align with that vision.

- **Choose to opt out** of diet talk and body-shaming conversations. Try to elevate the conversation by offering a compliment or lifting someone up.

- **When you're tempted** to make a negative comment about your body, swap it out for a positive statement or redirect your thoughts toward something you're grateful for.

- **When there are ups and downs** on your journey, don't be surprised and don't beat yourself up. Be kind to yourself, and choose grace over guilt. And remember you can start fresh week after week, day after day, hour after hour.

Vision Guide

Use the following questions and reflections to help you to evaluate where you are now.

1. On a scale of 1 to 10, how do I currently feel about the way I am taking care of myself?

   ....

2. What's working well in my health, fitness, and self-care routine?

   ....

   ....

   ....

   ....

3. What's not working well?

   ....

   ....

   ....

   ....

4. Why is taking care of my health important to me?

   ....

   ....

   ....

   ....

▶▶

Now take a moment to create a vision for who you want to be and how you want to care for your health in the future. Write your answers in the present tense, as if you've already attained them.

1. Each day, I feel . . .

2. I take care of my mental and physical health by . . .

3. When things don't go as planned, I . . .

4. When I get to the end of each day, I . . .

As I move forward, I will embrace progress over perfection, choose grace over guilt, and celebrate progress, no matter how small.

Acknowledgments

This book would not exist without the help and support of so many wonderful, wise, and brilliant people.

First and foremost, to the Lindywell community: thank you. Without your support and shared passion for this mission, this book would not exist. I am so grateful for each and every one of you. Bringing this book to life was a true team effort, and I couldn't have done it without the amazing women on the Lindywell team.

Becky, where do I even begin? Thank you for paying attention to every detail and keeping me on track. Your insight and wisdom are threaded into every page of this book.

Angie, I'm still pinching myself! From our very first conversation on your deck to your creative vision, branding, and leadership, your eye for beauty and expression helped bring this book to life. It would not be what it is without you. Thank you for pushing me.

To every other member of the Lindywell team—you know who you are—thank you for bringing this book to the world and for believing in our vision and purpose with so much heart and passion. I am so grateful for each of you.

To my incredible agent, Jenni Burke: thank you for seeing the potential in me and the power in this message. Your guidance, support, and friendship have been a gift to me since the day we first met. I feel like I won the lottery when I met you!

To the entire Tyndale Refresh team: Jan, Jillian, Kristen, Libby, Dean, and everyone behind the scenes. Thank you for believing in me and this book and for helping bring this vision to life. Stephanie, your support in every sentence of this book was a gift. Thank you for your encouragement and wisdom as I worked through each word, each sentence, and each paragraph.

And lastly, to Matt and my kids: thank you for your unending support and love—for letting me sneak away to write these pages and for providing the encouragement I needed to keep going. I am forever grateful.

Notes

CHAPTER 1: REFRAME

1. R. P. Abernathy and D. R. Black, "Healthy Body Weights: An Alternative Perspective," *American Journal of Clinical Nutrition* 63, no. 3 (March 1996): 448S–451S, https://academic.oup.com/ajcn/article/63/3/448S/4651512.
2. Tracy L. Tylka et al., "The Weight-Inclusive versus Weight-Normative Approach to Health: Evaluating the Evidence for Prioritizing Well-Being over Weight Loss," *Journal of Obesity* (July 23, 2014): 983495, https://www.hindawi.com/journals/jobe/2014/983495/.
3. "Wellness Industry Statistics and Facts," Global Wellness Institute, accessed September 24, 2022, https://globalwellnessinstitute.org/press-room/statistics-and-facts.
4. B. J. Fogg, *Tiny Habits: The Small Changes That Change Everything* (Boston: Houghton Mifflin Harcourt, 2020), chap. 6.
5. Tiffany A. Ito et al., "Negative Information Weighs More Heavily on the Brain: The Negativity Bias in Evaluative Categorizations," *Journal of Personality and Social Psychology* 75, no. 4 (1998): 887–900, https://pubmed.ncbi.nlm.nih.gov/9825526/.
6. Brené Brown, *I Thought It Was Just Me (but It Isn't): Telling the Truth about Perfectionism, Inadequacy, and Power* (New York: Gotham Books, 2008), 197.
7. Anne Craig, "Discovery of 'Thought Worms' Opens Window to the Mind," Queen's Gazette, Queen's University, July 13, 2020, https://www.queensu.ca/gazette/stories/discovery-thought-worms-opens-window-mind.
8. Kristin Neff, *Self-Compassion: Stop Beating Yourself Up and Leave Insecurity Behind* (New York: William Morrow, 2011).

CHAPTER 2: MOVE

1. Simply visit lindywell.com to start a free trial of at-home Pilates workouts you can do in less than twenty minutes a day.
2. Sang Hwan Kim et al., "Mind-Body Practices for Posttraumatic Stress Disorder," *Journal of Investigative Medicine* 61, no. 5 (June 2013): 827–834, https://pubmed.ncbi.nlm.nih.gov/23609463/.
3. Lidia Zylowska et al., "Mindfulness Meditation Training in Adults and Adolescents with ADHD: A Feasibility Study," *Journal of Attention Disorders* 11, no. 6 (May 2008): 737–746, https://pubmed.ncbi.nlm.nih.gov/18025249/.
4. Joseph H. Pilates and William John Miller, *Pilates' Return to Life through Contrology* (New York: J. J. Augustin, 1945), 12.
5. Joseph H. Pilates and William John Miller, *Pilates' Return to Life through Contrology*, rev. ed. (Ashland, OH: Presentation Dynamics, 2012).

6. Bessel van der Kolk, *The Body Keeps the Score: Brain, Mind, and Body in the Healing of Trauma* (New York: Penguin Books, 2015), chap. 5.

7. B. J. Fogg, *Tiny Habits: The Small Changes That Change Everything* (Boston: Houghton Mifflin Harcourt, 2020), 2.

8. Min Zhao et al., "Beneficial Associations of Low and Large Doses of Leisure Time Physical Activity with All-Cause, Cardiovascular Disease and Cancer Mortality: A National Cohort Study of 88,140 US Adults," *British Journal of Sports Medicine* 53, no. 22 (2019): 1405–1411, https://pubmed .ncbi.nlm.nih.gov/30890520/.

9. Kelly D. Brownell and Judith Rodin, "Medical, Metabolic, and Psychological Effects of Weight Cycling," *Archives of Internal Medicine* 154, no. 12 (June 27, 1994): 1325–1330, https://pubmed .ncbi.nlm.nih.gov/8002684/.

CHAPTER 3: NOURISH

1. Tim Peterson, "Healthspan Is More Important than Lifespan, So Why Don't More People Know about It?" Institute for Public Health, May 30, 2017, https://publichealth.wustl.edu/healthspan -is-more-important-than-lifespan-so-why-dont-more-people-know-about-it/.

2. Stuart Wolpert, "Dieting Does Not Work, UCLA Researchers Report," UCLA Newsroom, UCLA, April 3, 2007, https://newsroom.ucla.edu/releases/Dieting-Does-Not-Work-UCLA-Researchers-7832; A. D. Higginson and J. M. McNamara, "An Adaptive Response to Uncertainty Can Lead to Weight Gain during Dieting Attempts," *Evolution, Medicine, and Public Health* 2016, no. 1 (January 2016): 369–380, https://academic.oup.com/emph/ article/2016/1/369/2803021; Kelley Strohacker, Katie C. Carpenter, and Brian K. McFarlin, "Consequences of Weight Cycling: An Increase in Disease Risk?" *International Journal of Exercise Science* 2, no. 3 (July 15, 2009): 191–201, https://europepmc.org/article/MED/25429313.

3. Roma Pahwa, Amandeep Goyal, and Ishwarlal Jialal, "Chronic Inflammation," in *StatPearls* (Treasure Island, FL: StatPearls Publishing, January 2022), last updated June 19, 2022, https://www.ncbi.nlm.nih.gov/books/NBK493173/.

4. David Furman et al., "Chronic Inflammation in the Etiology of Disease across the Life Span," *Nature Medicine* 25, no. 12 (December 2019): 1822–1832, https://www.nature.com/articles /s41591-019-0675-0.

5. Lilli Link, "Are You Inflamed? 5 Signs to Look Out For," Parsley Health, March 21, 2018, https://www.parsleyhealth.com/blog/5-signs-chronic-inflammation/.

6. Margriet S. Westerterp-Plantenga, Sofie G. Lemmens, and Klaas R. Westerterp, "Dietary Protein— Its Role in Satiety, Energetics, Weight Loss and Health," *British Journal of Nutrition* 108, no. S2 (August 2012): S105–S112, https://pubmed.ncbi.nlm.nih.gov/23107521/.

7. "Food Marketing to Children," State of Childhood Obesity, accessed September 28, 2022, https://stateofchildhoodobesity.org/policy/food-marketing-to-children/.

8. Jessie Inchauspé, *Glucose Revolution: The Life-Changing Power of Balancing Your Blood Sugar* (New York: Simon and Schuster, 2022), xvii.

9. "Food Deserts," Food Empowerment Project, accessed September 28, 2022, https://foodispower .org/access-health/food-deserts/.

10. "The Water in You: Water and the Human Body," Water Science School, US Geological Survey, May 22, 2019, https://www.usgs.gov/special-topics/water-science-school/science/water-you -water-and-human-body.

11. Douglas S. Kalman et al., "Comparison of Coconut Water and a Carbohydrate-Electrolyte Sport Drink on Measures of Hydration and Physical Performance in Exercise-Trained Men," *Journal of*

the *International Society of Sports Nutrition* 9, no. 1 (January 18, 2012): 1, https://www.ncbi.nlm
.nih.gov/pmc/articles/PMC3293068/.

CHAPTER 4: LISTEN

1. E. E. Hill et al., "Exercise and Circulating Cortisol Levels: The Intensity Threshold Effect," *Journal of Endocrinological Investigation* 31, no. 7 (July 2008): 587–591, https://pubmed.ncbi.nlm.nih .gov/18787373/.
2. Zhaowei Kong et al., "Short-Term High-Intensity Interval Training on Body Composition and Blood Glucose in Overweight and Obese Young Women," *Journal of Diabetes Research* 2016 (September 20, 2016): 1–9, https://pubmed.ncbi.nlm.nih.gov/27774458/.
3. Tunde K. Szivak et al., "Adrenal Cortical Responses to High-Intensity, Short Rest, Resistance Exercise in Men and Women," *Journal of Strength and Conditioning Research* 27, no. 3 (March 2013): 748–760, https://pubmed.ncbi.nlm.nih.gov/22561973/.
4. Bessel van der Kolk, *The Body Keeps the Score: Brain, Mind, and Body in the Healing of Trauma* (New York: Penguin Books, 2015), 274.

CHAPTER 5: UNPLUG

1. L. Ceci, "Average Time Spent Daily on a Smartphone in the United States 2021," Statista, June 14, 2022, https://www.statista.com/statistics/1224510/time-spent-per-day-on-smartphone-us/.
2. K. R. Subramanian, "Myth and Mystery of Shrinking Attention Span," *International Journal of Trend in Research and Development* 5, no. 3 (June 2018), http://www.ijtrd.com/papers/IJTRD16531.pdf.
3. Yehuda Wacks and Aviv M. Weinstein, "Excessive Smartphone Use Is Associated with Health Problems in Adolescents and Young Adults," *Frontiers in Psychiatry* 12 (May 28, 2021), https://www.frontiersin.org/articles/10.3389/fpsyt.2021.669042/full.
4. American Friends of Tel Aviv University, "Heavy Cell Phone Use Linked to Oxidative Stress," ScienceDaily, July 29, 2013, www.sciencedaily.com/releases/2013/07/130729133531.htm.
5. "Health Risks of Using Mobile Phones," South University, August 10, 2016, https:// www.southuniversity.edu/news-and-blogs/2016/08/health-risks-of-using-mobile -phones-137310.
6. Sehar Shoukat, "Cell Phone Addiction and Psychological and Physiological Health in Adolescents," *EXCLI Journal* 18 (February 4, 2019): 47–50, https://www.ncbi.nlm.nih.gov /pmc/articles/PMC6449671/.
7. Cal Newport, *Digital Minimalism: Choosing a Focused Life in a Noisy World* (New York: Portfolio /Penguin, 2019), 108.
8. "Circadian Rhythms," National Institute of General Medical Sciences, last updated May 4, 2022, https://www.nigms.nih.gov/education/fact-sheets/Pages/circadian-rhythms.aspx.
9. Liese Exelmans and Jan Van den Bulck, "Bedtime Mobile Phone Use and Sleep in Adults," *Social Science and Medicine* 148 (January 2016): 93–101, https://pubmed.ncbi.nlm.nih.gov/26688552/.
10. Stephen M. James et al., "Shift Work: Disrupted Circadian Rhythms and Sleep—Implications for Health and Well-Being," *Current Sleep Medicine Reports* 3, no. 2 (June 2017): 104–112, https://pubmed.ncbi.nlm.nih.gov/29057204/.
11. Lucy E. Keniger et al., "What Are the Benefits of Interacting with Nature?" *International Journal of Environmental Research and Public Health* 10, no. 3 (March 6, 2013): 913–935, https:// www.mdpi.com/1660-4601/10/3/913/htm.
12. Nipith Charoenngam and Michael F. Holick, "Immunologic Effects of Vitamin D on Human Health and Disease," *Nutrients* 12, no. 7 (July 15, 2020): 2097, https://www.mdpi.com/2072-6643/12/7/2097.
13. Rebecca Burton, "Sunlight Gives Energy to Infection-Fighting T Cells," April 27, 2017, in *Health in*

a Heartbeat, UF Health Podcasts, 1:59, https://podcasts.ufhealth.org/sunlight-gives-energy-to -infection-fighting-t-cells/.

14. Winfried E. H. Blum, Sophie Zechmeister-Boltenstern, and Katharina M. Keiblinger, "Does Soil Contribute to the Human Gut Microbiome?" *Microorganisms* 7, no. 9 (August 23, 2019): 287, https://www.mdpi.com/2076-2607/7/9/287.

15. Ronald D. Hills Jr. et al., "Gut Microbiome: Profound Implications for Diet and Disease," *Nutrients* 11, no. 7 (July 16, 2019): 1613, https://www.mdpi.com/2072-6643/11/7/1613.

16. Bum-Jin Park et al., "Physiological Effects of Shinrin-yoku (Taking in the Atmosphere of the Forest)—Using Salivary Cortisol and Cerebral Activity as Indicators," *Journal of Physiological Anthropology* 26, no. 2 (March 2007): 123–128, https://pubmed.ncbi.nlm.nih.gov/17435354/.

17. Gaétan Chevalier et al., "Earthing: Health Implications of Reconnecting the Human Body to the Earth's Surface Electrons," *Journal of Environmental and Public Health* 2012 (January 12, 2012): 291541, https://www.ncbi.nlm.nih.gov/pmc/articles/PMC3265077/.

CHAPTER 6: CONNECT

1. Roger O'Sullivan et al., "Impact of the COVID-19 Pandemic on Loneliness and Social Isolation: A Multi-Country Study," *International Journal of Environmental Research and Public Health* 18, no. 19 (September 23, 2021): 9982, https://www.mdpi.com/1660-4601/18/19/9982/htm.

2. Debra Umberson and Jennifer Karas Montez, "Social Relationships and Health: A Flashpoint for Health Policy," *Journal of Health and Social Behavior* 51, no. S1 (2010): S54–S66, https://journals .sagepub.com/doi/10.1177/0022146510383501.

3. Kendra Cherry, "What Is a Collectivist Culture?" Verywell Mind, updated February 23, 2022, https://www.verywellmind.com/what-are-collectivistic-cultures-2794962.

4. Umberson and Montez, "Social Relationships."

5. Brené Brown, "The Power of Vulnerability," TEDxHouston talk, October 6, 2010, video, 20:44, https://www.youtube.com/watch?v=X4Qm9cGRub0.

CHAPTER 7: REST

1. Björn Rasch and Jan Born, "About Sleep's Role in Memory," *Physiological Reviews* 93, no. 2 (April 1, 2013): 681–766, https://pubmed.ncbi.nlm.nih.gov/23589831; Banner Health, "How Sleep Can Affect Stress," February 28, 2019, https://www.bannerhealth.com/healthcareblog/teach-me /how-sleep-can-affect-stress.

2. "Good Sleep for Good Health," News in Health, National Institutes of Health, April 2021, https://newsinhealth.nih.gov/2021/04/good-sleep-good-health.

3. Joseph A. Hanson and Martin R. Huecker, "Sleep Deprivation," in *StatPearls* (Treasure Island, FL: StatPearls Publishing, 2022), last updated June 21, 2022, https://www.ncbi.nlm.nih.gov/books /NBK547676/.

4. Wenyu Huang et al., "Circadian Rhythms, Sleep, and Metabolism," *Journal of Clinical Investigation* 121, no. 6 (June 1, 2011): 2133–2141, https://www.jci.org/articles/view/46043.

5. Brett A. Dolezal et al., "Interrelationship between Sleep and Exercise: A Systematic Review," *Advances in Preventive Medicine* 2017 (March 26, 2017): 1364387, https://www.ncbi.nlm.nih .gov/pmc/articles/PMC5385214/.

6. A. J. Metz et al., "Continuous Coloured Light Altered Human Brain Haemodynamics and Oxygenation Assessed by Systemic Physiology Augmented Functional Near-Infrared Spectroscopy," *Scientific Reports* 7 (August 30, 2017): 10027, https://www.nature.com/articles /s41598-017-09970-z.

7. Daniela Litscher et al., "The Influence of New Colored Light Stimulation Methods on Heart Rate Variability, Temperature, and Well-Being: Results of a Pilot Study in Humans," *Evidence-Based Complementary and Alternative Medicine* 2013 (November 28, 2013): 674183, https://pubmed.ncbi.nlm.nih.gov/24369481/.

8. Margareta Asp, "Rest: A Health-Related Phenomenon and Concept In Caring Science," *Global Qualitative Nursing Research* 2 (April 29, 2015): 2333393615583663, https://www.ncbi.nlm.nih.gov/pmc/articles/PMC5342845/.

9. "Relaxation," Women in Balance Institute, accessed October 8, 2022, https://womeninbalance.org/lifestyle-strategies/relaxation.

10. Judith E. Carroll et al., "Partial Sleep Deprivation Activates the DNA Damage Response (DDR) and the Senescence-Associated Secretory Phenotype (SASP) in Aged Adult Humans," *Brain, Behavior, and Immunity* 51 (January 2016): 223–229, https://pubmed.ncbi.nlm.nih.gov/26336034/.

11. "Why Downtime Is Essential for Brain Health," Cleveland Clinic, June 2, 2020, https://health.clevelandclinic.org/why-downtime-is-essential-for-brain-health.

12. Risa Kagan et al., "Impact of Sleep Disturbances on Employment and Work Productivity among Midlife Women in the US SWAN Database: A Brief Report," *Menopause* 28, no. 10 (August 30, 2021): 1176–1180, https://pubmed.ncbi.nlm.nih.gov/34469936/; "The Importance of Rest and Relaxation," My Home Vitality, accessed October 8, 2022, https://www.myhomevitality.com/how-rest-and-relaxation-can-make-you-more-productive.

13. Joanna York, "Why It's So Hard for US Workers to Ask for Time Off," Worklife, BBC, December 13, 2021, https://www.bbc.com/worklife/article/20211209-why-its-so-hard-for-some-workers-to-ask-for-time-off.

CHAPTER 8: BREATHE

1. Joseph H. Pilates and William John Miller, *Return to Life through Contrology* (New York: J. J. Augustin), 8.

2. James Nestor, *Breath: The New Science of a Lost Art* (New York: Riverhead Books, 2020), xix.

3. Andrea Zaccaro et al., "How Breath-Control Can Change Your Life: A Systematic Review on Psycho-Physiological Correlates of Slow Breathing," *Frontiers in Human Neuroscience* 12 (September 7, 2018): 353, https://pubmed.ncbi.nlm.nih.gov/30245619/.

4. Xiao Ma et al., "The Effect of Diaphragmatic Breathing on Attention, Negative Affect and Stress in Healthy Adults," *Frontiers in Psychology* 8 (June 6, 2017): 874, https://pubmed.ncbi.nlm.nih.gov/28626434/.

5. Hamayun Zafar et al., "Effect of Different Head-Neck Postures on the Respiratory Function in Healthy Males," *BioMed Research International* 2018 (July 12, 2018): 4518269, https://pubmed.ncbi.nlm.nih.gov/30112389/.

6. Linda Stone, "Just Breathe: Building the Case for Email Apnea," HuffPost, updated November 17, 2011, https://www.huffpost.com/entry/just-breathe-building-the_b_85651; Megan Rose Dickey, "Freaky: Your Breathing Patterns Change When You Read Email," Insider, December 5, 2012, https://www.businessinsider.com/email-apnea-how-email-change-breathing-2012-12.

7. Ma, "Effect of Diaphragmatic Breathing."

8. P. McKeown and M. Macaluso, "Mouth Breathing: Physical, Mental and Emotional Consequences," Oral Health, March 9, 2017, https://www.oralhealthgroup.com/features/mouth-breathing-physical-mental-emotional-consequences/.

9. "The Benefits of Breathing through Your Nose," Breathing and Sleep Center of Colorado Springs, September 2, 2020, https://breathingandsleepcenter.com/2020/09/the-benefits-of-breathing-through-your-nose/.

10. Sigrid Breit et al., "Vagus Nerve as Modulator of the Brain-Gut Axis in Psychiatric and Inflammatory Disorders," *Frontiers in Psychiatry* 9 (March 13, 2018): 44, https://pubmed.ncbi.nlm.nih.gov/29593576/.

11. Daniel B. Levinson et al., "A Mind You Can Count On: Validating Breath Counting as a Behavioral Measure of Mindfulness," *Frontiers in Psychology* 5 (October 24, 2014): 1202, https://pubmed.ncbi.nlm.nih.gov/25386148/.

CHAPTER 9: PLAY

1. "Building Better Mental Health," Help Guide, accessed October 25, 2022 https://www.helpguide.org/articles/mental-health/building-better-mental-health.htm.

2. Cale D. Magnuson and Lynn A. Barnett, "The Playful Advantage: How Playfulness Enhances Coping with Stress," *Leisure Sciences* 35, no. 2 (March 20, 2013): 129–144, https://psycnet.apa.org/record/2013-10188-003.

3. Lynn Barnett, quoted in Jennifer Wallace, "Play Is Important for Adults, Too," *Ledger* May 20, 2017, https://www.theledger.com/story/entertainment/recreation-activities/2017/05/21/play-is-important-for-adults-too/20827704007/.

4. René T. Proyer, "The Well-Being of Playful Adults: Adult Playfulness, Subjective Well-Being, Physical Well-Being, and the Pursuit of Enjoyable Activities," *Europeun Journal of Humour Research* 1, no. 1 (March 31, 2013): 84–98, https://www.europeanjournalofhumour.org/ejhr/article/view/Rene%20Proyer.

5. Joan Tupponce, "Laughter Relaxes the Body and Mind," *Richmond Times-Dispatch*, January 13, 2013, https://richmond.com/life/health/article_1db0eb92-5d13-11e2-891b-001a4bcf6878.html.

6. Mi Youn Cha and Hae Sook Hong, "Effect and Path Analysis of Laughter Therapy on Serotonin, Depression and Quality of Life in Middle-Aged Women," *Journal of Korean Academy of Nursing* 45, no. 2 (April 2015): 221–230, https://pubmed.ncbi.nlm.nih.gov/25947184/.

7. T. Matsuzaki et al., "Mirthful Laughter Differentially Affects Serum Pro- and Anti-Inflammatory Cytokine Levels Depending on the Level of Disease Activity in Patients with Rheumatoid Arthritis," *Rheumatology* (Oxford) 45, no. 2 (February 2006): 182–186, https://pubmed.ncbi.nlm.nih.gov/16319105/.

CHAPTER 10: CHOOSE

1. Eva M. Krockow, "How Many Decisions Do We Make Each Day?" *Psychology Today*, September 27, 2018, https://www.psychologytoday.com/us/blog/stretching-theory/201809/how-many-decisions-do-we-make-each-day.

2. Courtney E. Ackerman, "What Is Neuroplasticity? A Psychologist Explains [+14 Tools]," PositivePsychology.com, updated September 12, 2022, https://positivepsychology.com/neuroplasticity/.

3. Anne Trafton, "Distinctive Brain Pattern Helps Habits Form," MIT News, Massachusetts Institute of Technology, February 8, 2018, https://news.mit.edu/2018/distinctive-brain-pattern-helps-habits-form-0208.

4. Nikhil Swaminathan, "Why Does the Brain Need So Much Power?" *Scientific American*, April 29, 2008, https://www.scientificamerican.com/article/why-does-the-brain-need-s/.

5. B. J. Fogg, *Tiny Habits: The Small Changes That Change Everything* (Boston: Houghton Mifflin and Harcourt, 2020), chap. 5.

6. Rene Dailey et al., "The Buddy Benefit: Increasing the Effectiveness of an Employee-Targeted Weight-Loss Program," *Journal of Health Communication*, 23, no. 3 (2018): 272–280, https://pubmed.ncbi.nlm.nih.gov/29452062/.

About the Author

Like so many women, **Robin Long** struggled with body image and her on-and-off relationship with diet and workout programs. She wondered why she and other women work so hard to "fix their bodies," yet always feel disconnected from them. As she started to explore the question further, she realized she couldn't remember a time when she felt good in her body. She knew there was something deeper that needed to be explored.

It took a step inside the Pilates studio for Robin to change her entire approach to wellness. Pilates helped Robin connect her mind and her body for the first time. She started working with her body, not against it.

Robin's health and mental transformation motivated her to pursue a comprehensive Pilates certification through Body Arts and Science International, and ultimately perfect her own method of teaching Pilates—with a special focus on not just the body but also the mind.

After years of working with a constant three-month private training wait list, she knew she had to find a new approach to her practice. In order to help more people, she launched one of the very first online Pilates platforms, making Pilates more accessible to people around the world. Beginning with a blog, she brought her unique way of teaching online and made it accessible to anyone who wanted to learn a different approach to whole-body wellness.

What started out as Robin teaching private clients more than twelve years ago has turned into a global wellness platform that reaches millions of women in more than a hundred countries around the world.

As founder and CEO of Lindywell, Robin still loves to create classes and programs that transform her clients and members from the inside out. She lives in sunny Santa Barbara, California, with her husband, Matt, and their four children.

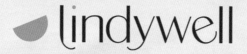

lindywell

A realistic and sustainable approach to getting fit and feeling good for a lifetime

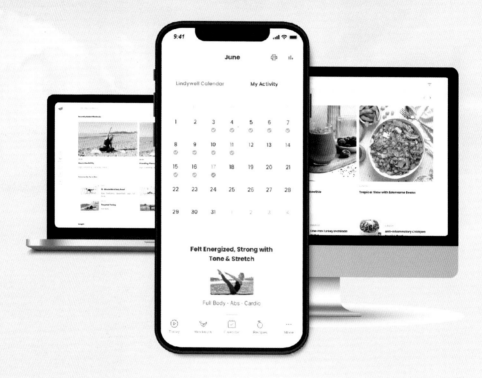

Join our community for access to strength-building Pilates workouts, restorative breathwork sessions, and nourishing recipes to reduce inflammation and increase your energy.

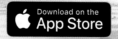 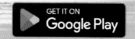

Learn more at Lindywell.com

CP1911